Nicklaus Children's Hospital

MIAMI CHILDREN'S HEALTH SYSTEM

ÜNITED for Patient Safety

PATIENT SAFETY AWARENESS WEEK

Jane— thought you might be interested in this history — Andy

March 12–18, 2017

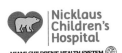

Hospice Care for Children

Hospice Care
for Children

EDITED BY

Ann Armstrong-Dailey
Sarah Zarbock Goltzer

New York   Oxford
OXFORD UNIVERSITY PRESS
1993

Oxford University Press

Oxford   New York   Toronto
Delhi   Bombay   Calcutta   Madras   Karachi
Kuala Lumpur   Singapore   Hong Kong   Tokyo
Nairobi   Dar es Salaam   Cape Town
Melbourne   Auckland   Madrid

and associated companies in
Berlin   Ibadan

Copyright © 1993 by Oxford University Press, Inc.

Published by Oxford University Press, Inc.,
200 Madison Avenue, New York, New York 10016

Library of Congress Cataloging-in-Publication Data
Hospice care for children / edited by Ann Armstrong-Dailey, Sarah
Zarbock Goltzer.
p.   cm.
Includes bibliographical references and index.
ISBN 0-19-507312-6
1. Terminally ill children—care.   2. Hospice care.   3. Terminally
ill children—Family relationships.   I. Armstrong-Dailey, Ann.
II. Goltzer, Sarah Zarbock.
[DNLM: 1. Attitude to Death.   2. Grief.   3. Hospice Care—in
infancy & childhood.   4. Hospices—organization & administration.
WS 200 H8284]
RJ249.H69   1993
362.1'75—dc20
DNLM/DLC
for Library of Congress   92-48937

9 8 7 6 5 4 3 2 1

Printed in the United States of America
on acid-free paper

To my children and theirs,
and to all of my family who carry
the torch handed down by G. G.

A. A. D.

To my dad, James W. Zarbock.
I am both proud and blessed to know that
the apple does not fall far from the tree.

S. Z. G.

FOREWORD

C. Everett Koop, M.D.
Former U.S. Surgeon General

Children's hospice care is a concept of care that can take place in a hospital, at home, or other residential care setting. Having worked with dying children for 35 years, I confess to an experience-based preference to permit children to die at home in the center of a loving family. This home-centered care also offers the family a cost-effective alternative to hospital care. Through the efforts of persons, such as yourselves, who are committed to meeting the special needs of children with life-threatening conditions and their families, public and professional awareness is heightened. Each of the disciplines that will benefit from reading *Hospice Care for Children* has a role and responsibility for continuing to enrich that circle of care.

Children are not immune to serious illness and death. Most parents of these children want involvement and some control over their children's care. In addition, the emotional strain and grief faced by these families is overwhelming, often leading to increased incidence of job loss, alcoholism, and drug abuse.

As a pediatrician and as a father who has lost a son, the importance of children's hospice care is especially clear. The grief felt at such a time is one unlike any other, the pain and loss immeasurable. As stated in my memoirs, nothing changed our lives—and the lives of our surviving children—like the death of our son, David.

Children's hospice care can make a difference. It facilitates the participation of parents in assuming the role of primary caregiver. It supports the inclusion of the patient and the family in the decision-making process to the best of the family's capability and commensurate with their desires. This comprehensive care can have a lasting impact on the lives of family members and friends, making it possible to find some solace and comfort mixed among the grief.

PREFACE

Children are not supposed to die. But they do. Approximately 100,000 children die each year in the United States alone. An estimated 7 million children worldwide are seriously chronically ill.

Timmy, a 5-year-old child with nephrotic syndrome, spent his last few weeks of life in a leading children's hospital. When his prognosis was terminal, he was moved to a room at the end of the hall. Timmy's health-care providers, feeling failure and denial, and his parents, unable to bring themselves to face his inevitable death, withdrew from him emotionally. Timmy blamed himself and tried to understand what he had done to drive everyone away.

Timmy died without physical pain but emotionally isolated, without the reassurance of his parents' love. To paraphrase Mother Theresa: The greatest pain on earth is not the pain of hunger or poverty but rather the pain of isolation, abandonment, and feeling unloved. Through hospice-type support, Timmy, his parents, and his health-care providers could have known what they were feeling was normal. They could have cried together and expressed how they would miss one another. They could have shared the picture of the butterfly, bearing the words, "I Love You, Mom," which Timmy drew just before he died, alone.

The loss of a child can be a devastating experience for the family. Children's hospice care can turn this potentially destructive experience into a strengthening and bonding one for the family. The knowledge that you have done everything possible for your child can be of great comfort.

Health-care providers, trained to cure, encounter their own unique challenges when a child they are involved with dies. The concept of children's hospice care, incorporated into their regimen, reminds health-care providers that they can continue to "care" even when they cannot "cure." Staff support programs ensure that they receive appropriate support themselves.

Children's hospice care has been developed to meet the special needs of children and their families facing death situations. It is a concept of care bringing together physicians, nurses, social workers, therapists, teachers, clergy, administrators, and volunteers as a team to provide the care and support needed. The child and family are the leaders of the team. The focus of hospice care is on life and living—improving the quality of life for the patient and the ongoing lives of the family.

Children's Hospice International (CHI) was founded in 1983 as a non-profit organization to provide resources and support to children with life-threatening conditions and their families, and to provide education, training, and technical assistance to health-care professionals.

CHI is a living memorial to Alan H. Armstrong. The sudden loss of my brother, Alan, following the death of my parents, was devastating—when such an integral part of your life is removed, all that is seemingly important falls away. With Alan's death, however, he gave me the greatest gift of all—an understanding of how truly important every day is, and a knowledge that what we choose to do with each day matters greatly.

This book can be a useful tool in enabling you to touch the lives of the children and families you serve. The death of a child is perhaps the most difficult to bear. As Abraham Lincoln noted—you have not known grief until you have stood at the grave of your child. Death and serious illness profoundly impact the lives of those they touch. Each of us must effect what change we can to ensure that it is not a lasting negative influence. The difference is yours to make.

Alexandria, Va.   A.A.D.
November 1992

ACKNOWLEDGMENTS

The production of this comprehensive book on children's hospice care is a landmark event. It is a project that would not have been possible without the untiring work of Sarah Zarbock Goltzer, Joan Bossert, Terri Southwick, Esq., and each of the chapter authors.

The inspiration for this book comes from children with life-threatening conditions, families facing the death of a child, and from the health-care providers who care for them—those who focus us on life and living, and on the quality of every child's life and the ongoing life of the family.

My personal inspiration came from my grandparents, G. G. and V. T. Rice who, having buried four of their five children and one grandchild, still managed to live life to its fullest. They taught us by example how to turn pain into positive action.

Many have dedicated themselves to caring for children and families, establishing the groundwork on which children's hospice care was built. Children's Hospice International (CHI) augments the work of these leaders who include: Mother Theresa, Elisabeth Kübler-Ross, M.D., C. Everett Koop, M.D., Rabbi Earl A. Grollman, Ph.D., Antonia Novello, M.D., Dame Cicely Saunders, Josephina Magno, M.D., The American Academy of Pediatrics, The National Association of Children's Hospitals and Related Institutions, The National Hospice Organization, and organizations of the United Nations.

For their early leadership in the field, we commend the Hospice of Northern Virginia, Edmarc, Children's Hospital of Milwaukee, Helen House, Children's Hospital of Los Angeles, San Diego Hospice, Oakland Children's Hospital, Hospice of West Palm Beach, Hospital for Sick Children, St. Mary's Hospital for Children, Children's Hospital National Medical Center, Johns Hopkins Children's Center, and the Royal Alexandria Hospital for Children.

In recent years, the importance of international cooperation on health-care issues has been recognized. Thanks to international organizations, collaborative efforts, and the growing interest of a number of nations, the needs of children and families worldwide will be better met. Children's hospice care meets a growing need, and the children's hospice movement has evolved to meet the demand. To the many individuals and organizations who have been part of this movement and who are committed to the provision of this care, thank you.

I'd like to express personal gratitude to Phil Pizzo, M.D. — an inspiration to us all showing us the importance of caring even in our desperate fight to cure; to Barbara Bush, Senator Robert Dole, and Senator Claiborne Pell, who have pledged their ongoing support to children's hospice care; to Arthur Kohrman, M.D., Harry Jennison, M.D., Robert Sweeney, Bernard A. Nigro, M.D., and Richard Huberman, M.D., who recognized the need for and who have provided ongoing support for CHI since the early years; to Patricia Dailey — daughter, friend, and "right arm"; to Robert A. Milch, M.D. — friend, mentor, and continued inspiration; to the dedication and support of Pat McCulla, the Board of Directors, staff, and volunteers of CHI; to Patrick Grant, Esq., and Vivian Berzinski, Esq., of Arnold & Porter, and to Woody Britain and Richard Larkin of Price Waterhouse, for pro bono legal, organizational, and financial counsel.

May the loving memories of Melinda Lawrence and Bill Reinecke be reflected in the ongoing care of children with life-threatening conditions, and their families. Most important, special thanks to all those we serve, who continue to be our best teachers.

A.D.D.

A number of individuals have been instrumental in the development and completion of this book. My special thanks and gratitude go to my co-editor for her continued support and wise counsel and her total dedication to the cause; Giulio D'Angio, M.D., for his unwavering faith in what I have wanted to accomplish, both at Children's Hospital of Philadelphia and in the creation of this book; Joan Bossert, our Oxford editor, for her persistence, patience, and enthusiasm; my family, for their ongoing encouragement and love, and especially my mother, for giving me the benefit of her extensive knowledge and talent for writing and critiquing (and gardening); to Randi Wirth, for helping me to get to where I wanted to go; to all of the authors, who devoted their considerable time and energy; and to Charlotte and Isadora, for always being there.

S.Z.G.

CONTENTS

III Appendix

CONTRIBUTORS

Ann Armstrong-Dailey
Children's Hospice International
Alexandria, Virginia

Paul R. Brenner
Montgomery Hospice Society
Rockville, Maryland

Charles A. Corr
School of Humanities
Southern Illinois University at
  Edwardsville
Edwardsville, Illinois

Betty Davies
School of Nursing
University of British Columbia;
Research Division
British Columbia Children's
  Hospital
Vancouver, British Columbia
Canada

Cindy Fair
Social Work Department
The Clinical Center
National Institutes of Health
Washington, D.C.

Kathleen W. Faulkner
Pediatric Hematologist-
  Oncologist
Dover, Massachusetts

Martha Blechar Gibbons
University of Maryland School of
  Nursing
Department of Maternal-Child
  Health
Baltimore, Maryland

Sarah Zarbock Goltzer
Medical Writer/Editor
Wayne, Pennsylvania

Ellen Gortler
Maryland Infants and Toddlers
  Program
Governor's Office for Children,
  Youth, and Families
Baltimore, Maryland

Bernice Catherine Harper
Health Care Financing Adminis-
  tration
Department of Health and Human
  Services
Washington, D.C.

Doris A. Howell
Department of Pediatrics
University of California, San Diego
La Jolla, California

C. Everett Koop
Senior Scholar
C. Everett Koop Institute at
  Dartmouth
Hanover, New Hampshire

Neil Lombardi
Medical Services
St. Mary's Hospital for Children
Bayside, New York

Ida Martinson
School of Nursing
Department of Family Health Care
  Nursing
University of California, San
  Francisco
San Francisco, California

xvi

Angela W. Miser
Department of Anesthesiology
University of Washington School of
  Medicine
Seattle, Washington

James S. Miser
Department of Pediatrics
University of Washington School of
  Medicine
Seattle, Washington

James R. Monahan
Hospice of Central Florida, Inc.
Maitland, Florida

Cheryl Marco Naulty
Walter Reed Army Medical
  Center
Department of Pediatrics
Washington, D.C.

Philip A. Pizzo
Pediatric Branch
National Cancer Institute
Bethesda, Maryland

Julie Simpson Sligh
Edmarc Hospice for Children
Portsmouth, Virginia

Andrew R. Tartler
Family Continuity Programs
St. Petersburg, Florida

Lori Wiener
Pediatric Branch
National Cancer Institute
Bethesda, Maryland

J. William Worden
Department of Psychology
Rosemead Graduate School of
  Psychology
LaMirada, California

Hospice Care for Children

Introduction

Hospice is a special form of comprehensive care provided to people who have a serious, progressive illness as well as to their families. The purpose of hospice care is to enable these patients and families to live as fully and comfortably as possible, by providing pain and symptom control as well as physical, psychologic, emotional, and spiritual support services.

The concept of hospice has its roots in the Middle Ages, when Crusaders, weary from their journey, were offered safe haven in way stations. Monastic orders also offered a refuge for traveling pilgrims, where individuals could find shelter, food, and companionship and visit with others who were on a religious quest. The concept of hospice today is applied to patients who are traveling through the final stages of their lives—in effect, seeking shelter and comfort. Hospice encompasses death as just one part of the continuum of life.

It was Dame Cicely Saunders, an English physician, who first developed the idea of physical and emotional support for dying patients. In 1967, based on the hospice model of Calvary Hospital in New York City, Dr. Saunders opened and became the medical director of St. Christopher's inpatient hospice in London.

In the mid-1960s, when Saunders had the opportunity to lecture at Yale University's schools of medicine and nursing, several of her American colleagues became interested in creating a similar program of hospice care in New Haven. In 1974, funded by the National Cancer Institute as part of a three-year demonstration project, these individuals developed the first American hospice home care program.

A critical aspect of early hospice care was the absolute need to provide patients relief from their pain, focusing first and foremost on prevention. Saunder's work and the hospice movement overall were reinforced by the research and teachings of Dr. Elisabeth Kübler-Ross, as put forth in her landmark book, *On Death and Dying*, first published in 1969. Today there are more than 1700 hospices in this country as part of both hospitals and home health agencies, as well as in free-standing and skilled nursing facilities.

The concept of pediatric hospice care is a natural extension of the hospice philosophy as it has already been applied to adults. Although hospice planners initially focused on adults because of their larger numbers, it became increasingly apparent that there was a need for children's hospice care as well. One of the earliest advocates, Dr. Earl Grollman, addressed children's special needs in *Explaining Death to Children*, published in 1956. In the early 1970s, a home care program for children with cancer was one of the first models used in the development of future pediatric hospice programs. But progress was slow. In fact, by 1983, of the approximately 1400 hospice programs in the United States, only 4 were able to accept children as patients.

Modeling themselves on adult hospices and recognizing that hospice is a philosophy not a facility, other models of pediatric hospice gradually developed and included care delivered in different settings. Early leaders in providing children's hospice services were Edmarc, a community-based hospice home care program in Virginia, which first started caring for children in 1979; Hospice of Northern Virginia, the first adult-oriented home care program to develop a children's component in 1979; St. Mary's Hospital for Children, a comprehensive inpatient palliative care program in Bayside, New York, started in 1985; and Helen House, an inpatient program providing respite care only, started in Oxford, England in 1982.

As the need for hospice care for children became better appreciated, more adult hospices included children in their programs. As part of this effort, Children's Hospice International, a nonprofit organization founded in 1983, had three goals: (1) to encourage the inclusion of children in existing and developing hospice home care programs; (2) to include the hospice philosophy in all areas of pediatric care, education, and the public arena; and (3) to promote hospice support through pediatric care facilities. By 1985, 183 hospices accepted children and as of 1989, 447 hospice programs provided care to children. Today over 1000 hospices are willing to consider accepting children into their programs.

It has been said that the quality of a civilization can be judged by how well it takes care of its elderly; this same comment can be applied equally to how well we care for our children, especially those with life-threatening or terminal illnesses. The access to and provision of hospice care for children is increasing, as more professionals from a wide variety of disciplines as well as the general public begin to appreciate the need and value of treatment and support services for this special pediatric population and their families. Unfortunately, denial that a child will die, on the part of both professional caregivers and loved ones, although quite understandable, remains a major obstacle to getting appropriate and effective intervention for those who need it, when they need it.

Hospice Care for Children is a compilation of national and international authorities in the field of pediatric hospice and offers a theoretical background for each of the individual components of care, but, more important, it offers practical information and recommendations about how and where to get this specialized care.

The first part, "Issues in Clinical Management," provides specific information about providing care for this group of children. Topics include children's age-related understanding of death, the critical elements of pain and symptom control, and the psychosocial aspects of life-threatening illnesses in childhood and adolescence. The unique issues of neonatal death and caring for the child with HIV infection and AIDS are also described.

Caring for the dying child has a profound effect on many others. Part II, "Support Systems," addresses the needs of the family, special school programs for children and their classmates, the pain of siblings, and how to care for bereaved parents. The child's primary physician, other professional staff, and specially trained volunteers also play uniquely important roles and require their own emotional support.

There is no one *right* way to develop a pediatric hospice program. Each location has different needs, resources, and patient demographics. The Appendix includes information about pediatric hospices in three separate settings and covers the experiences of Edmarc Hospice for Children, the Home Care for the Child with Cancer nursing research study in Minnesota, and the inpatient Palliative Care Unit at St. Mary's Hospital for Children. Also located in the Appendix is an annotated bibliography of the wide variety of children's literature on death, and additional resources including grief periodicals for adults and children as well as resources for educators and professional journals and associations.

This book is meant to be read, underlined, reread, and *used*. Jot down notes in the margin; follow up on some of the resources; contact the programs and experts and ask questions. You may not read all of the chapters, though information from a range of professional disciplines is provided here. However, we believe you will gain knowledge to enhance what you already know or will gather new information for useful applications.

Readers of this book will, we hope, help continue breaking down the barriers to care for these children and their families. We all have a valuable contribution to make. Start the journey by taking the time now to sit down and read your first chapter—not for our or even your own sake, but for the children.

PART I

Issues in Clinical Management

1

Children's Understanding of Death

KATHLEEN W. FAULKNER

Children understand death in a complex and evolutionary fashion that varies greatly from the way adults understand it. They begin their exploration of the meaning of death as toddlers. This occurs spontaneously and inevitably. As children acquire greater intellectual, social, and emotional capabilities, they apply these skills to develop an increasingly mature concept of death.

In the aggregate, children's understanding of death occurs in a surprisingly predictable fashion. At an early age, death, separation, and sleep are all entangled in children's minds. These concepts get sorted out, but children are still likely to feel that death can be caused by a wish; can be undone with a wave of a wand; and is distantly removed from their own families. As children grow, both their understanding and their questioning become more sophisticated. The dead cannot move, but can they see or dream? Old people die, but at what age do people become old? Death dramatically affects the individual, but how does it also affect society? Children use the bits and pieces of information they glean over the years to develop an increasingly sophisticated understanding.

There are large variations in the rate of acquiring a mature concept of death, which reflect individual children's experience and environment. Children's intellectual capabilities and emotional makeup, their personal experiences with death, their cultural and religious backgrounds, and the learning environment of the family are all factors that are inexorably entwined in their concept of death. This chapter will explore this evolutionary understanding of death and the factors that influence it.

COGNITIVE UNDERSTANDING

> When I was a child, I spoke as a child, I understood as a child, I thought
> as a child: but when I became a man, I put away childish things.
> For now we see through a glass darkly; but then face to face: now I
> know in part; but then shall I know even as also I am known.[1]

Most children learn to recognize when something is dead before they reach the age of 3. This recognition has been consistently documented using either the verbal approach of an open-ended interview,[2] or the nonverbal approach of asking children to select pictures of dead or sleeping animals.[3] Children do not need to directly experience a death in order to realize its existence, although they do incorporate their life experiences into their understanding of death.

In order to study the learning process, researchers have tended to divide the complicated concept of death into various components. An understanding of these subconcepts is helpful in appreciating and categorizing children's knowledge.

Definitions of the Components of a Death Concept

There are four components, or subconcepts, that children incorporate into their self-education about death. These are irreversibility, universality, nonfunctionality, and causality.

Irreversibility refers to the understanding that once people die, their bodies do not become alive again. This incorporates the notion that death is permanent, irrevocable, and final. To elicit children's knowledge of this component, a researcher might ask questions like "Can dead people came back to life?" or "How do you make dead things come back to life?"

Universality refers to the understanding that everyone will die. This includes the concept that people known to the child, or the children themselves, might die. Questions that might be asked include "Do all people die?" or "Will you die?"

Nonfunctionality refers to the cessation of life-defining processes. Included in this component are the lack of bodily functions. Questions exploring this component could include "What does it mean to be dead?" or "Can a dead person dream?"

Causality refers to identification of possible reasons that people die. It embraces external causes of death, internal causes of death, and sometimes the notion of suicide. Questions directed toward understanding this component could be "How do people die?" or "What can make people die?"

Ages versus Stages: Limitations of the Research

Having established the particular components to be studied, most researchers then attempt to correlate their subjects' responses with either the chronological age of the children or their level of cognitive development. There are now over fifty studies of children's understanding of death, and a pattern of acquisition of knowledge does emerge. There are disturbingly marked variations in this pattern, however, that need to be addressed before adopting a global scheme of "normal" development.

Undoubtedly, methodological variations in the research account for much of the discrepancy in results. These are well considered in Speece and Brent's comprehensive review of forty published papers on the topic.[4] They point out the difficulties in correlating the available studies. In some cases the sample size was small and did not include a full age-range of children. Many had sample populations limited to white, middle-class, suburban children. The standardized interview was the most frequently used technique to elicit information from children about their understanding of death, but the difficulty and specificity of the questions varied considerably. Some investigators explored nonverbal communication of information, ranging from drawings, to descriptions of death-related pictures, to spontaneous or directed play. With few exceptions, these efforts could not be standardized between studies. There was no consensus regarding statistical analysis of the results.

Besides methodological limitations, efforts to develop a global theory have been hampered by the question of how best to define the markedly different phases that children go through in the evolvement of their concept of death. The definition has tended to be either age-based or stage-based on Piaget's general theory of cognitive development.[5]

The age of the child is undoubtedly an important factor. Both Kane and Orbach found internal consistency in their large sample populations between the age of the child and the development of death subconcepts.[3,6]

A child's level of cognitive development is broadly linked to an understanding of the various components of an understanding of death in many studies that have evaluated this theory.[3,7] Complete concordance has been lacking in some studies, however.[8] Part of the difficulty is that Piaget did not look directly at the way children learn about death. Therefore researchers have had to extrapolate which cognitive skills children need in order to acquire each of the components of a mature concept of death.

By using both children's ages and their levels of cognitive development, it is possible to reach a consensus on how children as a group interpret death at various points in their childhood. Following recognition of death, they pass through consistent phases in the way they define death. These have been well outlined by Kane and others.[3]

Children start by identifying the structure of death. They concentrate on what it looks like to be dead. They then begin to appreciate the effect of death on function. This begins with an exploration of its effects on bodily function and progresses to include effects on the mind and spirit. Finally, they grow to a phase where they are able to consider the abstract implications of death. This includes a visualization of their own death, and the effect of death on other people and society as a whole.

Despite knowing how children as a group learn to understand death, the age and cognitive phase of an individual child cannot be used to assume that particular child's understanding of death. So far that information can only be obtained by personal communication with the individual child about the subject of death.

Given these limitations, it is still helpful for the hospice worker to know the general phases that children pass through on their way to an adult concept of death.

The Separation Phase

The separation phase encompasses children from birth to 3 years of age and embraces the sensorimotor stage of Piaget. Children in this phase are unlikely to differentiate death from temporary separation or from abandonment.

Since the verbal skills of this group are limited, their concerns are chiefly expressed through crying, separation anxiety, and attachment to the primary caregiver. The need for close and continuous physical contact in this age group is paramount. The end of this phase is marked by the realization of death as a separate entity, and the development of a concept that defines death in terms of structure.

The Structural Phase

Defining death in terms of structure is found in predominately 3- to 6-year-old children in Piaget's preoperational thought stage. They recognize death in terms of lying-down immobility, but may not recognize that being dead and being alive are mutually exclusive. Thus death is often viewed as reversible and temporary. In this phase, children closely associate death with sleep or going on a trip. Children in the structural phase have fantasy reasoning and magical thinking. Belief in their ability to cause death by their thoughts or actions is indicative of their egocentric reasoning. They associate death with old age, but are uncertain about what is "old." They seldom have an appreciation for the possibility of their own deaths.

Children in this phase have concerns with death that center around separation, immobility, fear of sleep, and conflicts that arise when their internal realities are discrepant with external realities (i.e., a dead person does not return). Their potential for misplaced guilt is high. To allay these concerns requires continued physical contact, repeated reassurances, and gentle instruction toward a more mature understanding. When children begin to add functional considerations to their concept of death they are moving to the next phase.

The Functional Phase

Children in the functional phase are generally 6-to-12 and in Piaget's concrete operational stage. They are problem solvers, with the beginnings of logical thought. During the early years of this phase, children rapidly acquire a specific and concrete understanding of death. Thus by the age of 7, most children will have a concept of death that recognizes all the components of irreversibility, universality, nonfunctionality, and causality.[4] The components are held concurrently, without an attempt to interrelate them. Their understanding of the components enlarges and becomes more complex as they progress through this phase. Early on children list external causes of death; the possibility of internal causes are added later. They are fascinated by the specific details of death: decomposition, burials, and coffins. Children in the later part of this phase are able to envision their own deaths, although they continue to associate death most strongly with old age.

Children in the functional phase also continue to have concerns with isolation and separation. Additionally, they worry about body integrity and loss of control. In their struggle for "scientific" information they are vulnerable to acquiring confused or incorrect facts. Their verbal skills have improved dramatically, but they may be more interested in exploring their new bodily strength than talking. Children in this phase need to have their bodies treated with careful respect, to be offered specific factual information, and to have as much control over their situation as possible. They benefit by having nonverbal forms of communication (drawing, music, play therapy) made available to them. When children begin to interrelate the various components in their understanding of death, they are moving to the phase of abstract thinking.

The Abstract Phase

Children in this phase are generally aged 12 and up and are in Piaget's formal operations phase of cognitive development. Their thinking is consistent with reality and logical; in addition, they are able to speculate on the implications and ramifications of death. They now add to their complete definition of death the effect it has on other people and on society as a whole. In the heightened emotional period of adolescence, they can conceive of death as being "heroic" or "tragic." During this phase, children are very future oriented; so while they can conceive of their death in the future, it is generally difficult for them to appreciate as a present possibility.

Concerns of children in this phase center around a new awareness of their bodies and bodily image, and their reliance on peers for companionship and support. They are vacillating between a new awareness of the outside world and a continued need for the close support of a family. They may adopt acting-out or risk-taking behavior rather than approach a problem directly. Adolescents facing impending death may express anger by being medically noncompliant; fear by isolating themselves totally from peers; or sorrow at their loss of a future by wanting to marry.

Adolescents are best supported by realizing their needs as children while recognizing their developing adult skills. They need privacy without abandonment and the opportunity to interact with peers. They usually have a strong drive to document their lives in a global context, through the making of tapes, drawings, or writing stories. Maladaptive behavior needs to be recognized and appreciated for its underlying motives. And finally, they can be taught that the strong emotions of love and sorrow are part of adult life as well as childhood.

EMOTIONAL AND EXPERIENTIAL FACTORS

Given the global theory of how children come to appreciate the meaning of death, it is helpful to consider the factors that cause tremendous individual variations in understanding.

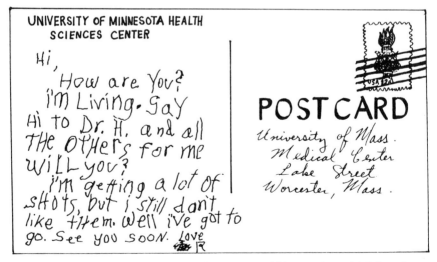

Figure 1.1 This postcard was written by a 9-year-old boy with Burkitt's lymphoma who was awaiting a bone marrow transplant.

Death Awareness in Life-Threatening Illness

As the above postcard depicts so graphically, having a life-threatening illness is one of the most powerful accelerators of a child's understanding of death. This message was written by a 9-year-old boy with Burkitt's lymphoma who was awaiting a bone marrow transplant. It combines the recognition of his own closeness to death and its significance for others found in a child in the abstract phase, with the matter-of-fact style and concrete concerns of a child in the functional phase.

The medical profession was slow to recognize that children with fatal illnesses were aware of their potential deaths. Much of the earlier literature on the subject was hampered by researchers' reluctance to gather information from the affected children themselves, relying instead on reports from parents or observers. Given children's extreme sensitivity to the affect of adults around them, it is easy to see, retrospectively, how a reluctance to listen could induce a reluctance to talk.

The open-minded observations of a few adults working with pediatric cancer patients led to the first controlled studies by Waechter and Spinetta looking at anxiety and awareness of death in these children.[9,10] They found that children with a potentially fatal illness had a much higher anxiety level in general, coupled with greater concern about body integrity, hospital personnel, and medical procedures. This was true whether or not they spoke openly about death; it was also true whether or not their life was immediately threatened. These findings are particularly revealing because the adults caring for these children, for the most part, did not speak about death to the children and maintained that the children were not aware of the fatal nature of their illness.

These high anxiety levels, feelings of isolation, and abstract fears have been identified as well in children around the world who suffer from a life-threatening illness.[11,12,13] The similarity of reports from cultures as disparate as Hungary, China, and England confirm that children are able to differentiate a potentially fatal illness from an acute or chronic nonfatal illness even in the absence of adult openness.

Death Experience

One of the most prominent ways that children with life-threatening illness learn the fatal nature of their disease is by experiencing the death of another patient.[14] Healthy children also have an accelerated understanding of death after experiencing the death of someone close to them or of multiple distant deaths. Several studies have shown that children who are "experienced" with death have more realistic data about death and the circumstances surrounding it and acquire the subconcept of universality at an earlier age. They are more aware of their own personal mortality.[3,15] This accelerated learning curve is much more pronounced in children less than 6 years of age who experience a death.

In modern society, the death of the family pet is often children's first exposure to loss and bereavement. This can be a powerful learning experience for children if adults do not minimize the grief.[16] Factual information about death can be shared, and the sometimes surprisingly strong emotions of loss and guilt can be faced together. Adults can help children devise appropriate rituals to commemorate the death. Additionally, the whole question of replacement of the dead animal can be discussed. Adults need to support children by allowing them time to grieve the dead pet. Yet they can also show that loving a new companion animal is not an expression of disloyalty to the dead pet. Instead it can be a reaffirmation of the value of the loving relationship between families and their animals. If granted validity by adults, the grief following a pet's death can introduce children to many of the concepts faced with human loss.

Effect of Disease and Treatment on Learning Ability

Many childhood life-threatening diseases now have chronic courses that can extend for many years. During this time, children's inherent ability to learn about death may be affected by either the disease or its treatment.

Pediatric acquired immunodeficiency disease (AIDS), for instance, has a strong neuropsychiatric component.[17] In the younger child, this may take the form of developmental delays, or actual loss of motor and verbal skills. Children with prenatally acquired AIDS may have had the additional risk of fetal alcohol or drug exposure. In the adolescent, psychoses and delirium may occur.

Current medical treatments may carry the risk of lessening children's cognitive abilities and interfering with their learning patterns. These effects have been seen in some forms of therapy directed against central nervous system leukemia in childhood,[18] for example.

Inherent Intellectual and Emotional Composition

Developing an understanding of death is a complex process that children accomplish privately over a number of years. It is not surprising, therefore, to find that children's individual intellectual abilities and emotional make-up influence that learning process. In general, more intelligent children acquire the various components of the concept of death at a younger age.[7,19]

High levels of generalized anxiety can slow the learning curve of even healthy, intelligent children.[19]

SOCIAL CONTEXT

> Death is not merely a biological phenomenon, but a social and
> cultural one as well.[14]

The search for complete comprehension of the meaning of death does not end when children reach adulthood. Throughout history, civilizations have grappled with the issue of placing death within the fabric of life in the society. This awareness has been accomplished through language, art, and song, and the establishment of elaborate death rituals and beliefs. Children will certainly be affected by the death culture of the society in which they live. They will also have their knowledge shaped by the immediate culture of their own family. These influences will combine with children's inherent beliefs and abilities to enrich their total understanding of death.

The Global Culture of Society

The research done in the past fifty years has given glimpses of how the global culture of the society in which children live affects their beliefs about death. One of the earliest studies done, that of Nagy interviewing Hungarian children, found that 5-to-9-year olds tended to personify death (i.e., the grim reaper, bogeyman).[2] This belief has seldom been replicated in other children in other cultures; however, Zweig also discovered a belief in a deathman in U.S. urban black children.[20]

Urban children, and children from lower socioeconomic backgrounds, are more likely to believe in external violence as a cause of death, whereas middle-class children will volunteer old age and ill health as prime causes.[20,21] Many have speculated on the effect of television-viewing on children's concepts about death. The often violent and grossly distorted image of death that is so prevalent on television might be expected to foster children's misconceptions. However, the one group of researchers who looked at this issue failed to document any specific distortions attributable to the amount or type of television exposure.[21]

The religious beliefs of children exert some influence over their understanding of death. This has been found to be true particularly in the areas of causation (i.e., people dying because they are "bad"), where children who are Catholic espouse this belief more often than whose who are Protestant, Jewish, or neither.[21] It also has an effect on the concept of life after death, where again the Catholic children held more strongly to this belief.

Even children who are not actively "religious" reflect society's ambivalence about whether death is a natural event or a punishment for some wrongdoing. In a study of children ages 5-to-9, White et al. found that, given a story about a mean old woman who died, the children were more likely to attribute her death to meanness rather than old age.[8]

The hospice caregiver needs to be attuned to these cross-cultural issues when caring for dying children and their families. This awareness may take additional effort to become educated about a culture's beliefs, religious structure, and methods of communication if the child and family is from a minority culture. Some of the critical differences have been outlined for Mexican and Vietnamese families, as well as inner-city black and Haitian families.[22,18] However, much work still remains to be done in this field.

The Immediate Culture of the Child's Family

Components that make up the child's family culture include all of the areas mentioned above: the race, nationality, and religious beliefs of the family and extended family. However, each family will vary in how completely it espouses the views of the global culture. The family's philosophical stance will be affected by previous experiences with death. Children's understanding of death within the family context will also be very much influenced by the patterns of communication that exist within that family. For children, it is not so important what their family believes, as how they feel about what they believe. Anxiety, avoidance, and fear are readily felt by children and can negate verbal reassurances of comfort with death.

It is important for caregivers to note that children are best supported within their family's cultural beliefs about death, even if these differ from the majority or those specifically of the caregiver. Attempts to change those beliefs as the family faces a life-threatening illness may make the eventual outcome less satisfactory for the family.[23]

COMMUNICATION WITH DYING CHILDREN

> And always understand that your real challenge is not just how to explain death to children, but how to make peace with it yourself.[24]

It is possible to know a child's age, level of cognitive ability, state of psychological health, sex, race, religion, socioeconomic status, nationality, experience with death, and family background. Even with all this information it is not possible to know what that child understands as death's meaning without approaching it (or letting the child approach it) directly. And, without this specific knowledge, it will be difficult to successfully relieve any anxieties or answer any questions that child might have.

Communicating with dying children about the subject of death has historically been difficult. In this century adults have become even less experienced because the number of deaths during childhood has declined dramatically. One hundred years ago, 50% of the deaths in the United States were composed of children younger than 15. Most parents had at least one child die before reaching adulthood. Today, less than 10% of those who die are children, leaving the adults caring for these children anxious and unskilled.

The implications for children facing a life-threatening illness are profound. In a classic study, Spinetta et al. documented the fatally ill child's growing sense of isolation from family and medical personnel.[25] A number of researchers have established that a pattern of open communication with the child can markedly reduce, though not eliminate, this psychological isolation.[9,23]

Sometimes with children, the best communication techniques are nonverbal ones. They benefit from an environment that is rich in opportunities to explore death, which can be done through dramatic play, art, music, puppetry, and even dance. All these forms of expressive therapy can allow children to demonstrate their needs and express their feelings and thoughts.[26]

Many children respond remarkably well to straightforward verbal communication. Nitschke et al. reported on the success of a "final-stage conference" held with all oncology patients older than 5 years, who were facing imminent death, and their families.[27] He found that the majority of the children understood their prognosis and wanted to be involved in the decisions regarding therapeutic options. Through all the research that has been done on communication with the dying child, there runs a theme that families rarely express regret in sharing too much information, but only too little.

When opening themselves to discussing death with children, adults need to follow guidelines to assure that children receive accurate and helpful information. Spinetta outlined salient points for medical caregivers to consider, and Adams gave guidelines directed toward parents.[23,28] To summarize these recommendations:

1. Follow children's leads regarding the timing and extent of communication. "Teachable moments" may be fleeting, and an immediate response may be necessary to capitalize on them.
2. Be specific and literal in explanations of concepts of death. Adult's euphemistic expressions surrounding death can be very confusing for children (i.e., equating death with sleep or a long trip).

3. Acknowledge the completeness of children's lives even if they are of brief duration. Help them find a sense of accomplishment and purpose, and let them know of their impact on their family and larger society.
4. Empower them as much as possible regarding the circumstances of their own death. Reassure them of continued love and physical closeness, of the absence of pain, and involve them in decisions that must be made.
5. Reassure children that a wide range of powerful emotions is appropriate when facing death. These can be expected from both children and adults.
6. Recognize when children need to be alone, as well as when they want to share. Children should not be coerced into talking about death; at times it may be more supportive to them to keep an element of hope alive.

The goal of communicating with the child who is dying is to meet the particular needs of that child. It is not necessary for children to have a mature understanding of death prior to their own deaths. However, correction of misconceptions, allayance of fears, and reduction of isolation will make the transition from life to death easier for the child. The dying child deserves always to be treated first as a child, and only secondarily as a dying person.

NOTES

1. 1 Corinthians 13:11–12. In *The Holy Bible, New King James Version* (1976). Nashville, TN: Thomas Nelson, p. 1123.
2. Nagy, M. (1948). The child's theories concerning death. J. Genet. Psychol. 73:3–27.
3. Kane, B. (1979). Children's concepts of death. J. Genet. Psychol. 134:141–153.
4. Speece, M.W., and Brent, S.B. (1984). Children's understanding of death: a review of three components of a death concept. Child Develop. 55:1671–1686.
5. Piaget, J. (1960). *The child's conception of the world.* New York: Littlefield, Adams.
6. Orbach, I., Talmon, O., Kedem, P., and Har-Even, D. (1987). Sequential patterns of five subconcepts of human and animal death in children. J. Amer. Acad. Child Adol. Psychiat. 26:578–582.
7. Koocher, G.P. (1974). Talking with children about death. Amer. J. Orthopsychiat. 44:404–411.
8. White, E., Elsom, B., and Prawat, R. (1978). Children's conceptions of death. Child Develop. 49:307–310.
9. Waechter, E. (1984). Dying children: patterns of coping. In Wass, H. and

Corr, C.A. (eds), *Childhood and death*. Washington, D.C.: Hemisphere, pp. 51–68.

10. Spinetta, J.J. (1974). The dying child's awareness of death: a review. Psychol. Bull. 81:256–260.

11. Polcz, A. (1981). Manifestations of death consciousness and the fear of death in children suffering from malignant disease. Acta Paediatr. Academ. Scien. Hungaricae 22:89–97.

12. Lee, P.W.H., Lieh-Mak, F., Hung, B.K.M., and Luk, S.L. (1983–84). Death anxiety in leukemic Chinese children. Intl. J. Psychiatry Med. 13:281–289.

13. Clunies-Ross, C., and Lansdown, R. (1988). Concepts of death, illness and isolation found in children with leukaemia. Child: care, health and development. 14:373–386.

14. Bluebond-Langer, M. (1978). *The private worlds of dying children*. Princeton, N.J.: Princeton University Press, p. 231.

15. Reilly, T.P., Hasazi, J.E., and Bond, L.A. (1983). Children's conceptions of death and personal mortality. J. Ped. Psychol. 8:21–31.

16. Robin, R., and ten Bensel, R. (1985). Pets and the socialization of children. In Sussman, M.B. (ed), *Pets and the family*. New York: Haworth Press, pp. 69–72.

17. Spiegel, L., and Mayers, A. (1991). Psychosocial aspects of AIDS in children and adolescents. Pediatr. Clin. North Am. 38:153–167.

18. Eiser, C. (1991). Cognitive deficits in children treated for leukaemia. Arch. Dis. Child. 66:164–168.

19. Orbach, I., Gross, Y., Laubman, H., and Berman, D. (1985). Children's perception of death in humans and animals as a function of age, anxiety and cognitive ability. J. Child Psychol. Psychiat. 26:453–463.

20. Zweig, A.R. (1983). Children's attitudes towards death. In Schowalter, J.E., Patterson, P.R., Tallmer, M., Kutscher, A.H., Gullo, S.V., and Peretz, D. (eds), *The Child and death*. New York: Columbia University Press, pp. 36–47.

21. McIntire, M.S., Angle, C.R., and Struempler, L.J. (1972). The concept of death in midwestern children and youth. Amer. J. Dis. Child. 123:527–532.

22. Spinetta, J.J. (1984). Measurement of family function, communication, and cultural effects. Cancer 53:2330–2338.

23. Spinetta, J.J., and Deasy-Spinetta, P. (1981). Talking with children who have a life-threatening illness. In Spinetta, J.J. and Deasy-Spinetta, P. (eds.), *Living with childhood cancer*. St. Louis, MO: C.V. Mosby, pp. 234–253.

24. Grollman, E.A. (1977). Explaining death to children. J. School Health 47: 336–339.

25. Spinetta, J.J., Rigler, D., and Karon, M. (1974). Personal space as a measure of a dying child's sense of isolation. J. Consulting Clinical Psychol. 42:751–756.

26. Schmitt, B.B., and Guzzino, M.H. (1985). Expressive therapy with children in crisis: a new avenue of communication. In Corr, C.A. and Corr, D.M. (eds.), *Hospice approaches to pediatric care*. New York: Springer, pp. 155–177.

27. Nitschke, R., Humphrey, G.B., Sexauer, C.L., Catron, B., Wunder, S., and Jay, S. (1982). Therapeutic choices made by patients with end-stage cancer. J. Pediatr. 101:471–476.

28. Adams, D.W., and Deveau, E.J. (1984). Children's knowledge of death. In *Coping with childhood cancer*. Reston, VA: Reston Publishing Company, pp. 139–152.

2

Pain and Symptom Control

JAMES S. MISER and ANGELA W. MISER

To take part in the care of dying children is a privilege. A strong commitment is required; the physical demands on the hospice team and the caregivers are sometimes draining; but the emotional and spiritual benefits to the individuals who care for dying children can build lasting strength.

THE ROLE OF PROFESSIONALS IN HOSPICE CARE OF CHILDREN: THE TEAM APPROACH

Because of the complexity of the problems that face a dying child and his family, it is critical that the team of medical professionals that cares for the dying child function well together and individually. At a minimum the team should consist of a physician, nurse, social work professional, and spiritual caregiver (chaplain, priest, or minister). All team members must view their relationship with the patient as equally important. To be effective the team must function together well but each individual must also have the strength and maturity to provide care separately.

The physician on the team must determine when the disease is refractory to conventional medical therapy and must be able to project accurately the potential risks and benefits of investigational therapy. By conveying this information accurately the physician will enable the child and the family to accept the dying process and to decide how long and how aggressively to pursue treatment of the primary disease.

Once the decision is made to no longer pursue curative therapy for the underlying disease, the primary role of the physician changes from a therapist of the disease to a provider of supportive care and effective symptom control to the child. This transition for the physician is difficult and often not made at all. However, to provide appropriate, necessary, and effective care to the child and the family, this transition must be made.[1,2,3,4] The commitment to the care of the dying child must be just as strong as the original commitment to treat the primary disease.

Children who are in a hospice setting often are dying because of a disease rather than due to an accident. Many of these diseases are complex and an intimate knowledge of the natural history of the disease by the physician is required to anticipate and diagnose the medical problems that will arise. Cancer, the most common cause of death due to disease, is a good example of this complexity. In the hospice setting, spread of cancer to new metastatic sites needs to be diagnosed early, with limited or no investigations, and with as much certainty as possible.

Although the physician need not be the captain of the hospice care team, he or she can effectively empower each member of the team by supporting each of them and by identifying and legitimizing the role of each team member with the family and child. As a child and family face death, many issues arise that go far beyond the physical death of the child. These emotional and spiritual issues can only be addressed adequately when the physical care issues are effectively managed. Conversely, when these emotional and spiritual issues are not addressed, the control of physical symptoms is more difficult.

The Importance of Maintaining Relationships

Strong relationships between people determine the quality of our lives. As many decisions are made in caring for the dying child, perhaps the most important factor to evaluate with each decision is the impact of the decision on the already established relationships that the child and the family have with each other, with friends and relatives, and with the medical and hospice professionals.

These relationships can intrinsically be therapeutic and can facilitate the acceptance of the supportive care that is required for managing symptoms effectively. Disruption of these relationships during the dying process can have a devastating effect on the quality of care and quality of life of the dying child. Simply maintaining contact with the dying child and the family by telephone can be successful if direct contact must be briefly interrupted. This strategy may be preferable to substituting an alternative caregiver even though the substitute may technically be as good. The broken relationship with the original caregiver may have lasting negative effects on the acceptance of care by the dying child and the family.

The dying process, if viewed as a dynamic part of life, is an opportunity to develop and to strengthen human and spiritual relationships, relationships of lasting benefit.

The Importance of Maintaining Dignity

Tom, a young boy of 8 dying of metastatic sarcoma, invited me in. I was making a home visit. As I entered, Tom was lying on the couch in the living room.

"Would you like something to drink?" he asked.

In most professional settings, I would normally have declined. However, it was clear that Tom's role as host meant a great deal to him. Having his doctor visit him at home was to him not primarily a medical appointment but a social visit.

"Thank you very much, Tom," I responded.

"We have Coke, orange juice, and a cup of coffee," he stated, clearly having prepared for the moment.

"I would be happy to have a cup of coffee, Tom," I said after some consideration.

"Mom, get Dr. Miser a cup of coffee," he commanded.

"Would you like cream in it?" he asked further.

"Thanks very much, I would," I again responded.

"Mom, don't forget to bring cream for Dr. Miser's coffee," he further directed. "Mom baked cookies, too. Would you like one?"

"Great. How are you, Tom?" I asked as I reluctantly began the task of assessing his physical condition after enjoying the social interaction.

Although dying and only able to lie quietly in his living room, Tom had been the perfect host and he was very pleased with himself. He had entertained his doctor. He had maintained his dignity. He had participated in the real stuff of life. While dying, he had done what he could for me. Knowing that the relationship was secure, signified by this sharing of refreshment, Tom subsequently accepted his doctor's care and his own condition.

Progressing and Achieving in the Dying Process

Progressing as an individual and achieving personal goals are possible and important during the dying process. Realistic goal setting that maintains the quality of life even though the quantity of activity must be reduced is an important component of a successful dying process. It is important for the hospice team to recognize that personal growth can be achieved during the dying process because the hospice team can promote and facilitate these personal goals. Most goals revolve around completing significant relationships with friends and relatives; however, experiential and spiritual goals are also not uncommon.

Said Mary, a teenaged girl from a Southern Baptist family, when told her cancer had recurred and was no longer responsive to chemotherapy, "Well, I guess there is nothing else to do except 'get saved'," she emphatically declared.

"I think you should do that," I supportively responded.

She scheduled her baptism for the next Saturday, was baptized, and died several weeks later.

Although dying young, a strong argument could be made that Mary achieved more spiritually in the last few weeks of her life than most of us do in a lifetime.

Thus, the death process can be one of dynamic personal growth and achievement.

The Importance of Attention to Detail

In delivering care a team can often become so involved in the process of team building and interaction that the details of care can be overlooked. It is sometimes assumed that the team is "taking care of things" when no single individual has taken the responsibility to make sure all the important details are addressed adequately. By attending to the very details of the physical, emotional, and spiritual aspects of the dying child's life, a peace and confidence can be achieved. If the child and the parents are absolutely confident that the team will address all the issues, they are relieved of the need to remember all the little questions that arise between visits. This attention to detail, more than anything else, convinces them that the team truly cares and will anticipate and solve problems.

PHYSICAL ENVIRONMENT

Much of the initial "set-up" of hospice care for the dying child relates to developing an appropriate physical environment. If the environment is optimal, the physical symptoms are both less in number and more easily controlled.

An important issue that must be addressed includes the kind of bed, which must be appropriate not only for the patient's medical condition but also for the emotional state of the child. Sometimes conflicts arise between the physical and emotional needs of dying children. A child may emotionally want to sleep in his own bed but may need the flexibility of a hospital bed. A child may emotionally want to be in the center of the action in the living room but needs the proximity to a bathroom or private commode. The successful resolution of these challenges defines successful management of the dying child. Depending on the medical condition, an air mattress, water mattress, or even more elaborate bedding may be required in order to equally distribute the body weight, thus avoiding skin breakdown. This is especially important when spinal cord involvement with tumor has resulted in denervation or when tumor blocks the circulation of an extremity resulting in progressive edema.

Where the child actually spends time is often not only dictated by the physical but also by the emotional needs of the child. Most children prefer to be at home for most or all of the dying process. Some request to go to the hospital just before death.

In the home, the child often has a variety of motives to change rooms: "to be in the middle of things" often results in moving to the living room; "to have privacy" often results in moving to a downstairs bedroom away from the front door and living room; "to be close to the family" often results in moving to the family room. Generally, the choice of where a child is to be and is to sleep should be determined after careful consideration of both the physical and emotional needs of the dying child and the family. However, if the child is in a desired space, symptom control will be considerably easier.

EMOTIONAL AND SPIRITUAL SUPPORT

The dying child will have better symptom control if the appropriate supportive emotional environment is provided. Maintaining normal relationships between the dying child and the family and friends and caregivers will have a dramatic effect on the child's life. Specifically, the control and prevention of symptoms is strongly related to the maintenance and growth of these supportive significant relationships.

Frequently, the question is asked by either father or mother, "Should I stay home from work to be with my dying child?" Although it may superficially seem obvious that the answer to this question is "Yes," before making such a decision, the effects on the relationships between parents and between each parent and the child should be considered. Often the lack of a normal "pattern of life" for at least one parent may have a significantly negative impact on the child and result in an increase in symptoms. This negative effect of bringing both parents together for an extended period under unusual circumstances must be balanced against the need to have the care of the dying child shared among all the significant caregivers. The "correct" solution may be different for each family and may change for each family from time to time. Here the hospice team can provide important counsel and support in these decisions. Importantly, the control of symptoms will be much more effective if all the "significant" relationships are intact.

A child and family that have a strong religious belief in God and belief in the power of God will often achieve peace in the midst of the dying process if their faith remains intact. Similarly, with spiritual support from family, church members, and friends their faith can actually grow in spite of the death of a child that is clearly not the will of God. Although the apparent spiritual conflict between what is God's will and what God allows plagues many parents who face the death of their child, those individuals with a strong faith and strong spiritual support will actually accept that they cannot know why the child must die without their faith being shaken.

The dying process, especially of a child, can precipitate a spiritual crisis for either the parents or the child that can then be reflected in physical manifestations and poorer symptom control. Effective spiritual support of these individuals can very often result in significant improvement in the control of the symptoms and in a more peaceful response to symptoms. Identifying those children and families in need of spiritual support is a key function of the hospice team.

For the older dying child who has had a spiritual experience, prayer is often a means of communication that results in a deeper relationship with God, a greater sense of spiritual peace, and a stronger sense of relationship with those around them. Thus, stronger relationships with God result in stronger spiritual relationships with others and stronger spiritual relationships result in improved emotional and physical relationships with others. All of these improved relationships result in improved symptom control.

The question often arises: "Who is the best person to provide the most effective emotional support?" The answer is everyone who has a significant relationship to the dying child and the family can and should provide emotional support within the context of their relationship with the dying child. The characteristics of this preexisting relationship in large part actually determine the degree of emotional support that can be provided by the individual. In extreme circumstances the health care team is called on to provide emotional support without these previously established relationships; however, this is often difficult and ineffective. Establishing relationships prior to the dying process almost always facilitates the delivery of subsequent health and supportive care. This is one of the primary advantages for the hospice team becoming involved early in the care of a dying child.

The importance of maintaining some of the "normal activities" cannot be overstated. Although the dying child will frequently be tired and will rest more than before, the desire to eat or participate in a favorite activity is maintained. Often there is only enough energy to begin a game, to play one hand of cards, or to eat one slice of pizza; however, participating brings dignity and self-esteem. The quality of each experience is much more important than the duration of each experience or the quantity of activity. These activities significantly enhance symptom control. For the participating normal family member or friend, realizing and coping with this "lack of stamina" may be extremely difficult. The individual with normal strength and stamina would usually say: "If we don't finish the game, what is the point? There really is no reason to start." The dying individual, however, will have fun and gain a sense of accomplishment in the participation even if completion is not possible. The role of the hospice team is to encourage both the dying child and those around him or her to participate in the activities of life even if the duration or the quantity of these activities do not seen "worth the effort." A strong sense of emotional well-being can be achieved if this participation is successfully accomplished.

SYMPTOM CONTROL

For a child in hospice care, the solutions for control of symptoms are not always the same as they are for the child who is undergoing active treatment for the malignancy. The major factor that obviates some symptomatic and supportive therapies is the inconvenience or the effort and energy required by the child to institute the therapy. A second major factor that obviates these therapies is the risk of side effects of additional supportive therapy. The third major factor that makes adding a new drug or therapy difficult is simply the requirement to change the therapy plan, even in a small way.

Changing doses, adding agents, and developing new plans must be done slowly and deliberately. Small gradual incremental changes in dosing are usually much better tolerated physically and emotionally than large increments followed by adjusting decrements.

As needed (PRN) medications are certainly required in the therapy plan of some dying children; however, PRN orders for frequently used drugs treating major symptoms such as pain are, in general, not effective and place the parent (or another caregiver) in the position of always having to judge whether and when the next dose of medication should be given. This continual reassessment usually results in much anxiety and loss of sleep. This approach also demands that a symptom or sign be exhibited before a PRN dose is to be given, that is, a child must have pain to receive pain medication. Because the goal of the hospice team is to prevent pain and symptoms completely, PRN medication orders should not be used when major symptoms are being treated and prevented. The alternative to medi-cating on a PRN basis is to use a fixed dose and schedule and to have a hospice team member reassess the treatment on a regular basis with the child and caregiver. Reassessing symptom control every two to three days is usually adequate if the child is relatively stable. Reassessing more fre-quently is necessary with a more rapidly evolving disease. This less fre-quent, scheduled reassessment gives the parent, caregiver, and child a sense of confidence that the child's condition will be evaluated with the hospice professional and that they will have input without the anxiety of constantly monitoring and deciding on the dose and the timing of each medication. The resulting improved sleep pattern for the child and parent often makes a major difference in the overall care.

Accurate diagnosis of new symptoms without invasive procedures, radio-graphic procedures, blood work, or cultures may be difficult in some cir-cumstances but can often be accomplished. Taking on this task is very important for the hospice team because better supportive care will result; however, the physician and hospice team must have an intimate knowledge of the natural history of the disease and an understanding of the physiologic changes that are taking place. This purely clinical diagnostic process re-quires even greater attention to detail than a diagnostic process supported by radiography and laboratory investigations.

Nausea and Vomiting

The specific cause of nausea and vomiting must be determined in order to most effectively treat this symptom of the dying child. Because the nausea or vomiting is not usually due to chemotherapy in this setting, but the disease itself or a side effect of one of the medications being given, strategies used successfully to prevent chemotherapy-induced emesis may not be as effective in this setting. Specifically ondansetron, a serotonin antagonist that is very effective in preventing chemotherapy-induced vomiting,[5,6] ap-pears not to be as effective in treating prolonged vomiting. Phenothia-zines (Thorazine) and lorazepam (Ativan) may be very effective in treating nausea and vomiting in the dying child; dexamethasone may also be benefi-cial.[6,7,8,9]

Vomiting may be a side effect of narcotics or other drugs including anti-biotics. It may also be due to physical conditions including increased intra-cranial pressure due to a central nervous system metastases, gastritis due to medications or stress, or a partial or complete bowel obstruction. Because the treatment of each of these causes of vomiting is very different, accurate rapid clinical diagnosis is essential. The nausea and vomiting due to narcotics are not infrequent and sometimes bothersome but usually not severe. Phenothiazines or lorazepam are often effective in treating narcotic-induced vomiting. The treatment of narcotic-induced vomiting occasionally requires a change to a different narcotic; however, a serotonin antagonist may also be tried. The vomiting due to metastatic central nervous system tumor is often abrupt and unaccompanied by nausea. It also may awaken the child out of sleep or occur in the early morning before ingestion of food. Dexamethasone and, if appropriate, cranial radiation are the treatments of choice for vomiting as a result of intracranial pressure due to tumor metastatic to the brain.

Vomiting due to gastritis can often be treated successfully by the combination of aggressive antacid therapy and a histamine (H_2) antagonist such as ranitidine. The vomiting due to partial or complete bowel obstructions usually must be primarily treated by decompression using nasogastric suction. Although surgical resection is occasionally indicated in a dying child, the usual treatment is ongoing decompression. Obstructions occasionally respond to pharmacologic therapy. Partial small bowel obstructions may be intermittent; however, in the terminal care setting the obstructions are often fixed and the symptoms unremitting.

In summary, the specific cause of the vomiting must be determined quickly by history and physical examination. Specific therapy must then be instituted to prevent this very unpleasant symptom.

Sleep Disturbances

Sleep disturbances are common in children who are dying. They often change their pattern of sleep either to a daytime sleeping and nighttime activity schedule or to an intermittent dozing pattern. Because both of these patterns can have a significant impact on the caregiver who usually still prefers a nighttime sleep pattern, establishing a regular nighttime pattern is preferable for most dying children and their families.

Emotional support and secure relationships are usually the main strategies to effect a more tolerable sleep pattern; however, medications are sometimes required. The potential interaction between these sedatives and the pain medications and other agents must be carefully anticipated. Chloral hydrate is the most common agent used; elavil can be of some benefit and can simplify medical management if it has other indications; phenothiazines (promethazine and thorazine) will often be effective if nighttime anxiety is the major cause of sleep disruption; lorazepam (Ativan) and triazolam (Halcion) are also beneficial. If the patient becomes confused and agitated, haloperidol (Haldol) and chlorpromazine (Thorazine) are frequently effective.

Anxiety

Anxiety is a frequent symptom in children who are dying. Moreover, anxiety frequently exacerbates other symptoms, especially pain. As discussed in an earlier section, strong relationships and excellent emotional and spiritual support are often the main therapeutic approaches to allay a child's anxiety in this setting. Further, the regular, dependable interaction with the hospice care professional also will allay much anxiety even if many of these interactions are only on the telephone. If these approaches do not work, medications can be given to treat anxiety. Phenothiazines (Thorazine) are usually the drugs of choice in children.[10] Benzodiazepines (Valium) may be used but often interact poorly and antagonistically with narcotics.[11] They frequently result in intermittent sedation and respiratory depression followed by anxiety on awakening when given simultaneously with narcotics. In contrast, it has been suggested that phenothiazines have a synergistic interaction with narcotics; they have been successfully used together with narcotics in pain cocktails. Thus, thorazine is usually the drug of choice when the child is already requiring narcotic analgesia.

Cardiorespiratory Symptoms

Cardiorespiratory symptoms are very frequent in dying children and may be due to direct involvement of the lungs by tumor, chronic lung disease due to chronic infections or prior therapy pneumonias, or cardiovascular deterioration caused most often by cardiomyopathy or progressive anemia. Occasionally upper airway obstruction can occur resulting in difficult to manage respiratory symptoms. The cause of cardiorespiratory deterioration must be determined accurately in order to implement effective therapy. At first patients may present only with an increased respiratory rate, but they may also have chest wall pain due to tumor invasion or to pleural effusion. Oxygen may not be required at first because the pathophysiology of many causes of respiratory disease is primarily restrictive and the body can maintain adequate ventilation with a compensatory increase in respiratory rate. Later when more disease is present, ventilation-perfusion inequalities occur, the restrictive disease advances, and hypoxia ensues. In contrast, some disease results in hypoxia early. Pneumonias, either due primarily to infections or primarily to an obstructive process, often present with hypoxia due to the ventilation-perfusion inequality. Because hypoxia also causes significant anxiety, it should be aggressively treated.

When cardiorespiratory deterioration is due primarily to cardiac dysfunction (heart failure) or progressive anemia, inadequate oxygen is being delivered to the tissues. Heart failure results in pulmonary edema which in turn results in hypoxia and significant anxiety. Oxygen, diuretics (furosemide), and sedation with morphine and phenothiazines will result in a much more peaceful respiratory pattern when pulmonary edema ensues. This less anxious pattern of respiration often results in a more effective oxygen exchange as well.[4,12]

Constipation

Although not apparently a major symptom, constipation can be a significant problem for the dying child. This symptom is also frequently focused on by the child and the family and must be dealt with successfully. Inactivity, narcotics, and poor oral intake predispose the dying child to a significant degree of functional constipation and abdominal pain. More serious causes of constipation include direct obstruction by tumor and neurologic involvement by tumor of the spinal cord or the sacral nerve roots.

Treatment of constipation should usually be pursued aggressively enough to prevent the accumulation of large amounts of stool and the development of pain.[13] For functional constipation, Colace, mineral oil, or Senokot can be combined in some pattern with effective results. Sometimes the addition of suppositories (Dulcolax) are also required. Enemas are usually not necessary but can have beneficial results in severe cases of constipation. For neurologically induced bowel dysfunction, stool softening, with care to avoid diarrhea, in conjunction with either gentle disimpaction or regular evacuation are necessary. The care of this neurologically induced problem is usually complicated by urinary denervation and paralysis of the lower extremities also due to the underlying neurologic compromise by the tumor.

Although radiation to the tumor involving the spinal cord or sacral roots is frequently given aggressively in patients early in the course of cancer treatment, it usually does not play a role in the child who is dying of cancer. Usually the difficult logistics and discomforts of administering radiation compared to the possible benefits results in a decision to pursue only supportive care without radiation. Nevertheless, each child and situation must be evaluated individually.

Urinary Dysfunction

Like constipation, urinary dysfunction can pose a significant problem for the dying child. Symptoms may include lower abdominal pain, dysuria, distension, frequency, enuresis, and hematuria. Urinary dysfunction, too, may become a major focus of the child and the family and thus must be dealt with effectively or the dying process may be significantly disrupted.

Inactivity, prior instrumentation, cachexia, obstruction by tumor, and the relative immunodeficiency of the cancer patient predisposes the dying child to an infection of the urinary tract (see below). Such an infection can become symptomatic and should be treated early.

Other common causes of urinary dysfunction include narcotic therapy for pain. More serious causes of urinary dysfunction include obstruction of the urinary tract by tumor and neurologic involvement by tumor of the spinal cord or the sacral nerve roots. As with treatment of bowel dysfunction due to neurologic involvement by tumor, radiation therapy is usually not pursued if the child is dying, most situations warranting only supportive care. When bladder function is lost, placement of a catheter may be required. Because maintaining dignity and relationships are very important issues for the dying child, avoiding a constant (or even frequent) odor of feces and urine is highly desirable and achievable. Inability to control these normal bodily functions resulting in "accidents," also has a significant impact on the child's self-esteem. As a result, a catheter is often the optimal choice to control urine when normal bladder function is lost. Generally, once the catheter is placed, it is well tolerated as long as it is carefully monitored and maintained by the team.

Once a catheter is placed the urine will become colonized with microorganisms; these need not be cultured for or treated unless the child becomes symptomatic (see "Urinary Tract Infections" below). Suppressive doses of antibiotics may be needed to prevent symptoms in some circumstances.

Infections

As part of planning the terminal care for a dying child a decision is often made to withhold antibiotics. Treating some infections with antibiotics, however, may significantly enhance the quality of life and the quality of relationships with the caregivers. As long as the purpose of the antibiotics is clearly to enhance the quality of the patient's life, they should be given. Even though superficially it may seem that the decision to withhold antibiotics would almost always seem the "correct course of action" because many patients die of infections and withholding antibiotics during the dying process is consistent with not intervening with death due to natural causes, antibiotics may significantly improve the patient's pain and discomfort during terminal care.

Urinary Tract Infections

Urinary tract infections can present with fever, lower abdominal pain, back pain, dysuria, frequency, and foul-smelling urine. All of these symptoms are disagreeable and have a deleterious effect on the dying child's quality of life. Clinical diagnosis without culture is often adequate in the hospice setting. Complicated circumstances may require cultures to determine the correct antibiotic therapy. Oral antibiotics are usually effective; occasionally, a brief course of parenteral antibiotics is preferred.

Cultures taken from the catheterized patient are frequently "positive." In spite of this colonization, treatment should generally be withheld until the patient is symptomatic as the antibiotics will have little lasting beneficial effect on the colonization and may, indeed, have a deleterious effect.

Pneumonia

Pneumonias are a common cause of death and, in general, are not treated aggressively once hospice care is chosen. A frequent cause of pneumonia is aspiration due to general inanition; other causes of pneumonia may include obstructive tumor or immunodeficiency. Occasionally, when the life expectancy is otherwise reasonably long and the child has some specific goals he wishes to achieve, a brief course of antibiotics to treat a limited aspiration pneumonia may be indicated. It is emphasized, however, that pulmonic processes are usually a significant component of the terminal event and, thus, intervention is usually not indicated except to prevent symptoms (i.e., oxygen and sedation).

Abscess

Occasionally the dying child may develop an abscess. Because these are frequently painful, antibiotic treatment and even incision and drainage under local anesthesia should be considered. Staphylococcal organisms are the most common causative microorganisms. Oral antibiotics are usually successful in this setting in controlling the spread of infection.

Fungal Infections

Dying children are predisposed to fungal infections for a variety of reasons including steroid therapy, antibiotic therapy, immunodeficiency, and neutropenia. Although the diagnosis of systemic fungal infections is not usually pursued in the hospice setting, superficial infections are not infrequent and can usually be treated easily and successfully. They are most commonly caused by *candida* species. Oral moniliasis (thrush) that may result in mouth pain can be simply treated with clotrimazole troches or mycostatin; superficial fungal skin infections, which occur most commonly in the perineal region, can be successfully controlled by mycostatin cream.

Fungating Tumor

Fortunately, primary tumor progression is a relatively uncommon event as a cause of death in children with cancer; however, when tumors become large and fungating, they can be very difficult problems. Their size, grotesque appearance, and repulsive smell may be particularly vexing. Fungating tumors not covered by skin do not have the usual host-defense mechanisms and barriers to infection. They can bleed, necrose, and become superficially infected, all of which lead to foul odors that can be embarrassing and repulsing. Superficial treatment and systemic therapy are both important.[4,14] Superficial therapy includes frequent dressing changes; Dakin's solution or acetic acid may be beneficial. Some wounds benefit from topical antibiotics such as topical application of 2% Clindamycin. Frequent cleaning with chlorhexidine (Hibiclens) may also be beneficial. Because these fungating tumors are frequently infected with anaerobic organisms (which cause a particularly putrid smell), treatment with a systemic antibiotic with anaerobic coverage is often useful. In this setting metronidazole (Flagyl) is the agent of choice.[4]

Skin[15]

Skin problems are common in children who are dying. Skin breakdown and superficial infections are the most common problems encountered and are caused by general malnutrition, resulting in weakness and lack of mobility, and by paralysis and denervation of the skin usually due to tumor involving the nervous system.

Although in many cases skin breakdown is inevitable, an appropriate bed and bed covering and clear instructions about how to prevent skin breakdown can avoid this problem. Once skin breakdown occurs, avoiding pressure and contact with the involved skin will prevent progression. Topical antibiotics may be necessary when superficial infections ensue. The most common site of skin breakdown is over the posterior iliosacral region; skin over the elbow and heels may also be affected. Elbow and heel "pads" can prevent skin breakdown in these regions.

Contractures

Contractures, especially of the lower extremities, are quite common in children who are dying. Predisposing causes include general lack of motion while in bed or denervation usually due to tumor involvement of the spinal cord or peripheral nervous system. Previous administration of neurotoxic agents, such as vincristine and cisplatin, may also contribute to this problem. The most common joint involved is the ankle. Once heel cord contractures occur, they are virtually impossible to correct; thus prevention is quite important. Since contractures will reduce what little mobility the child has, this will affect the child's sense of independence and dignity. Daily passive range of motion can usually prevent progression of contractures in the lower extremities and is something positive, physical, and nonpainful that the primary caregiver and the child can do together.

Neurologic Abnormalities

A variety of neurologic abnormalities may occur in a dying child. The most common include increased intracranial pressure, usually due to tumor within the brain; seizures; focal or generalized paralysis; and neuritic pain, usually from direct invasion by tumor.

Increased Intracranial Pressure

Increased intracranial pressure (ICP) is usually caused by primary or metastatic tumor within the brain. The symptoms of ICP include headache and vomiting which frequently occur in the morning or during the night causing arousal from sleep. Central nervous system involvement by tumor can also cause a variety of other neurologic manifestations including focal or generalized seizures, focal weakness, or spasticity.

In the hospice setting, ICP and its causes can be clinically diagnosed. Treatment with dexamethasone, four times daily is usually beneficial. Radiation therapy is generally not pursued in light of the patient's condition and the discomfort and inconvenience involved in administering radiation in this setting.

Seizures

Seizures may occur from a variety of causes including metabolic derangements of sodium, calcium, glucose, and magnesium; neurologic toxicity of drugs; and direct involvement of the central nervous system by tumor. Because seizures are particularly disruptive to the dying child and to his relationships with others and because seizures arouse a significant degree of fear, they should be controlled if at all possible. The drug of choice to treat seizures in this setting is diphenylhydantoin (Dilantin). Initial management requires a loading dose (usually intravenously) followed by regular oral dosing. If additional agents are required, phenobarbital or lorazepam are the agents of choice. Carbamazepine (Tegretol) may also be beneficial.

The importance of early clinical diagnosis and intervention without requiring supporting investigations (CT scans or EEGs) must be stressed.

Paralysis

Paralysis is usually due to the direct involvement of the nervous system, most often the spinal cord. This symptom is distressing and usually irreversible. Occasionally, dexamethasone will result in some improvement although it is usually transient. Because the diagnosis and treatment of the acute onset of paralysis in the hospice setting involves invasive procedures, is logistically difficult, potentially uncomfortable, disruptive, and inconvenient, supportive care is usually chosen. If the life expectancy of the child is still fairly long, radiation therapy may be useful, if introduced immediately. Invasive surgical decompression is rarely indicated in the hospice setting.

Neuropathic Pain

Direct involvement of the nerves by tumor may result in difficult to control neuropathic pain. This can also be caused by surgical denervation injury. Narcotics may be of some benefit, but frequently do not completely control neuropathic pain. Antidepressants (Elavil) and anticonvulsants (Dilantin, Tegretol) may be of significant benefit alone or in combination with narcotics.

Dehydration and Dry Mouth

Dehydration

Adequate hydration is sometimes difficult to achieve in dying children. Contributing factors to poor hydration include bowel dysfunction, an altered state of consciousness, mouth sores, difficulty swallowing, and nausea or vomiting. Inadequate hydration leads to a dry mouth and thirst. These are uncomfortable symptoms that should be avoided, if possible. In children, small amounts of fluid can usually be ingested frequently enough to avoid a dry mouth and maintain minimal urine output (½ to 1 cc per kilogram per hour). Because most children dying from cancer have central venous lines, intravenous maintenance fluids should be considered to avoid dehydration if oral hydration is not possible.

Dry Mouth

Dry mouth is often not due to dehydration but rather poor oral hygiene.[4] In addition to poor dental and mouth care, the most common causes of this problem in children are prior radiation, monilial infections, malnutrition, and drugs. Aggressive and frequent cleansing of the mouth including dental brushing, rinsing, and gentle debridement of necrotic ulcers is essential in managing this problem. Specific antibiotic therapy of fungal (thrush), bacterial (acute gingivitis), and viral (herpes simplex) infections should be instituted when these infections arise. Noninfectious acute mucositis is also occasionally seen. Topical anesthetics (viscous lidocaine, dyclonine) may provide some benefit for this problem but systemic narcotics are often necessary for moderate and severe cases.

It is very important to address this problem aggressively because the way a child's mouth feels, tastes, and smells may have a profound effect on how the child feels in general and how the caregivers and family relate to the child.

Nutrition

Progressive diseases, especially malignancies, cause a catabolic state, anorexia, malaise, and fevers that often result in progressive weight loss. The most common cause of weight loss in children, however, is decreased intake. Decreased intake may be due to emotional factors, systemic symptoms, mouth or mucosal pain, systemic or metabolic derangements, and as a side effect of narcotic therapy. Because weight loss is a distressing symptom for the patient and the parents, this issue must be addressed directly. The child will often be physically able to eat and drink only small amounts at each meal and, thus, small frequent feedings are often necessary. Hyperalimentation is usually not pursued. Although there is no absolute contraindication for hyperalimentation, it has not been established that hyperalimentation has measurable beneficial effects in dying children that would justify its risks, cost, and inconvenience. Other medical techniques used to stimulate the appetite in adults have been rarely attempted in children: corticosteroids, anabolic steroids, cyproheptadine (Periactin), and antidepressants. These therapies may be considered in specific circumstances.

PAIN CONTROL

Epidemiology

Pain experienced by dying children may be due to the underlying disease or its treatment. Much of the information about pain in dying children is gleaned from the experiences of children with cancer. Pain experienced by children with cancer may be cancer-related, treatment-related (e.g., mucositis, infection, radiation dermatitis, peripheral neuropathy, phantom limb, postoperative state), diagnostic/therapeutic procedure-related (e.g., venipuncture, bone marrow aspiration/biopsy, lumbar puncture), unrelated to cancer (e.g., trauma), or may arise from a combination of these causes.[16] Several surveys performed in single large institutions or in multi-institutional settings have documented that, unlike the experience in adults where reported pain is predominantly cancer-related,[17,18,19] ongoing pain experienced by children with cancer is predominately either therapy-related or unrelated to the malignancy, and that diagnostic/therapeutic procedure-related pain are almost universal causes of morbidity.[20]

When terminally ill patients alone are considered, one adult inpatient series indicated that 28% died without pain, while 72% required some form of analgesic management.[17] A second series, in which only adults dying with cancer pain were reported, documented that 77% had a combination of more than one type of pain.[21] Pediatric data are extremely sparse. However, Maunuksela et al.[22] followed the terminal course of 97 Finnish children with cancer who died during the period from 1983 to 1987. Of these, 44 were on active anticancer therapy at the time of death: 29 of 44 died without requiring pain management, many suffering a rapid demise from complications such as infections or hemorrhage. Of the 53 children dying while receiving supportive care alone, 28 required analgesia. No child in the five-year study period required analgesic treatment for more than six months, and 28 of the 40 children reporting pain required therapy for four weeks or less. This series complements the findings of others and displays the generally rapid demise once refractoriness to anticancer has occurred, and the significant morbidity caused by cancer treatment.

Since other series have documented, even in patients with active malignancy, that therapy-related pain is an important cause of morbidity,[16] the following features need to be considered when managing pain in terminally ill children: (1) the precise etiology of the pain should be documented wherever possible, since pain which is not directly cancer-derived is relatively common in this patient population and management of cancer-related pain, therapy-related pain, and unrelated pain may differ significantly; (2) once a childhood malignancy has become refractory to anticancer therapy, it is frequently rapidly progressive and generally requires close monitoring to achieve and maintain adequate pain control; (3) since invasive diagnostic therapeutic procedures are so commonly abhorred by children, the indication for performing each procedure should be carefully considered and, if deemed absolutely necessary, pediatric patients should receive optimal analgesic management to minimize the resulting pain and anxiety.

Adults have demonstrated that although oral analgesics frequently suffice for managing initial pain, an alternative route of drug administration is commonly required during the final days of life. Other symptoms, particularly fatigue, asthenia, sleepiness, and mental dysfunction, frequently accompany pain in terminally ill children, and should be anticipated and managed where possible.

Pain Syndromes

As in adults, invasion of bone and bone marrow are the commonest causes of direct cancer-related pain in children. Local bone destruction by primary tumors (e.g., osteogenic sarcoma or Ewing's sarcoma) or metastatic tumor usually gives rise to localized dull, aching, or boring pain. Rapidly expanding tumor, with or without associated intratumor hemorrhage, may result in sharp, excruciating pain. Vertebral involvement may likewise cause sharp, severe pain related both to bone invasion and paraspinal muscle spasm. Bone pain, which is severe, sharp, and markedly worse on movement, may be indicative of a pathologic fracture.

Invasion of the skull is particularly common in histiocytosis, neuroblastoma, and Ewing's sarcoma. Cranial vault invasion results in localized headache and may be accompanied by signs of raised intracranial pressure, if there is a significant intracranial extension. Invasion of the base of the skull, particularly common with rhabdomyosarcoma, leads to specific pain syndromes depending on location: retro-orbital, sinus, ear, and occipital pain from local tumor invasion are the most common. These are often associated with proptosis, bloody discharge from nose or ear, nasal obstruction, and cranial nerve palsies. Widespread bone marrow invasion, for example, in neuroblastoma or leukemia, is commonly associated with generalized severe aching limb and back pain.

Tumor invasion of the nervous system is also relatively common in the terminally ill child. Intracranial deposits of solid tumor result in signs and symptoms of raised intracranial pressure (severe headache and vomiting with early morning exacerbation) and associated neurologic deficits depending on tumor location. Raised intracranial pressure may occur from direct mass effect or from obstruction of cerebral spinal fluid pathways, particularly in the posterior fossa. Diffuse meningeal involvement, most frequent with leukemias and lymphomas but also seen with carcinomas and some brain tumors, results in raised intracranial pressure with or without the meningeal syndrome of back pain exacerbated by head flexion and straight leg raising. Localized spinal cord compression gives rise to local pain exacerbated by coughing, straining, straight leg raising, and neck flexion, tenderness to local percussion, paraspinal muscle spasm, and ultimately associated loss of neurological function (bladder dysfunction, sensory and motor dysfunction below the block). Referred pain may be experienced in the flank, groin, or anterior thigh due to upper lumbar cord compression or in the buttocks and posterior thigh due to lower lumbar cord lesions. Finally, compression of the long tracts in the cord may result in somewhat vague complaints of weakness, heaviness, or pain in the legs. Cord compression pain is perhaps the most critical syndrome to diagnose and manage as early as possible since delay will result in irreversible paralysis and a major decline in quality of life. Plexopathies, for example, of the lumbosacral plexus from sarcomatous invasion of the nerve trunk in the pelvis, results in local and/or radiating pain. Painful peripheral nerve invasion occurs infrequently but may arise from chest wall invasion of intercostal nerves or nerve entrapment over a tumorous bony prominence. Reflex sympathetic dystrophy[23,24] may occur occasionally and is most commonly associated with sarcomas of the pelvic or shoulder regions.

Soft tissue tumor involvement is frequently painless. Pain may occur from invasion of adjacent bone or nervous tissue; from obstruction of a hollow viscus (e.g., genitourinary rhabdomyosarcoma causing bladder neck or ureteral obstruction with resulting distention, colic, stasis, and infection); from obstruction of a drainage pathway (e.g., bronchus, biliary tree) leading to stasis and infection; from rapid tumor growth or intratumor hemorrhage leading to acute capsular distention (e.g., liver); from bowel invasion resulting in localized infection, partial or complete bowel obstruction, colicky abdominal pain, vomiting, perforation and peritonitis; and from tumor erosion of an intact mucosal surface leading to localized infection (e.g., fungating rhabdomyosarcoma of the nasopharynx, middle ear, or vagina). Localized infection may rapidly develop into generalized sepsis with shock in a child who is neutropenic from bone marrow invasion or following chemotherapy administration.

Evaluation

Before a management plan can be formulated, the following evaluation steps should be taken.

The Precise Etiology and Location of the Source of Pain Should Be Evaluated to a Degree Appropriate to the Clinical Status of the Child

At a minimum, an assessment of whether the pain is directly cancer-related or is related to therapy or an unrelated cause should be assessed since management strategies may be widely different between the broad categories. Some painful lesions, such as spinal cord compression and intracranial tumor deposits, require careful evaluation even in the child with very limited life expectancy because early intervention (for example, high-dose corticosteroid administration, irradiation) generally results in rapid pain relief and halting of progressive neurological compromise. Other pain syndromes may not require such careful diagnostic evaluation. For example, rapid development of multifocal bone pain from refractory neuroblastoma may best be managed with systemic analgesic drugs rather than irradiation to multiple sites, thus making a specific radiographic diagnosis of each new focus of bone pain unnecessary. With each new or progressive complaint of pain, the life expectancy of the child, the overall clinical status, and the most likely etiology of the pain need to be taken into consideration as the diagnostic evaluation is planned.

The Qualitative Features of the Pain and Overall
Pain Intensity Should Be Assessed

Qualitative features of pain[25,26,27] can be assessed only in children with sufficient verbal skills and prior experience with pain to adequately express what they are feeling. The assessment can, however, be extremely valuable in distinguishing, for example, the severe aching limb pain of relapsed leukemia from the burning hypesthesia and dysesthesia of a peripheral neuropathy.

An assessment of pain intensity should be made in every case.[28-42] Astute observations made over a period of time by an experienced health care professional or by a parent can be extremely valuable in assessing pain. In broad terms, the modalities available for pain assessment are changes in physiological parameters such as tachycardia, blood pressure elevation, and sweating; behavioral changes such as crying, moaning, grimacing, guarding, limping, overall withdrawal, and decreased movement and activity; age-appropriate patient self-report either by spontaneous description or using some form of intensity rating scale; and physical examination and laboratory evaluation where appropriate. In the terminally ill child, changes in physiological parameters cannot reliably be used as indicators of pain since they are affected by many other factors including infection and anemia. Likewise, many of the pain behaviors exhibited by an otherwise active, healthy child may be masked or absent in a child with severe anemia, infection, or major organ compromise. Many age-appropriate, formal patient-self-report, pain-intensity rating scales have been developed for use in children 3 years of age and older. Compliance with their use on a repeated basis can be problematic particularly in a sick child whose willingness to cooperate with even the simplest form of pain assessment may be severely compromised. The child who has previously been instructed in the use of one or more assessment scales prior to becoming terminally ill is the most likely to cooperate with the use of these tools since nothing new or unfamiliar is being demanded. The child unfamiliar with such assessment instruments may best be approached in the simplest of terms, such as a choice between "a little," "quite a lot," "a lot," "the worst" pain. Finally, physical examination for evidence of a painful lesion, questioning of parents and caregivers, and review of appropriate laboratory and radiographic parameters are essential in every case.

The Emotional State of the Family and Caregivers Should Be
Assessed in a Formal or Informal Manner

Major fears, anxiety, depression, interpersonal difficulties, spiritual needs, and unresolved issues of the dying process, where appropriate, should be assessed and addressed since each may have a major impact on pain management. In addition, financial stresses and the adequacy of the physical environment in which death will occur should be evaluated.

The Opinions of the Child and Family Regarding the Aggressiveness of Pain Management and Acceptable Analgesic Interventions Should Be Sought

For example, in a society in which children are taught to "say no to drugs," careful explanation of the appropriate medical use of analgesics may be appropriate, and the definitions of tolerance, physical dependence, and psychological dependence should be discussed.[43] *Tolerance* is a state in which increasing doses of a drug are needed to maintain the initial analgesic effect. Although the incidence and severity of tolerance to opioids during use in pediatric cancer patients is not known, this phenomenon undoubtedly occurs, particularly in children requiring parenteral opioid infusions for relief of severe pain. Fortunately, tolerance only occasionally causes a management problem since it can generally be managed by escalating the drug dosage as required. *Physical dependence* has occurred when sudden drug discontinuation or rapid dose reduction results in a well-characterized opioid withdrawal syndrome (e.g., tachycardia, "goose flesh," muscular jerks, abdominal pain, sweating, vomiting, diarrhea, flu-like symptoms, tremulousness, yawning, lacrimation, rhinorrhea, pupillary dilatation, and occasionally convulsions).[43] Withdrawal symptoms may be avoided by slowly tapering an opioid. *Psychological dependence* ("addiction") is characterized by craving the drug in question and by an overwhelming concern for obtaining and using it. This rarely, if ever, occurs following appropriate use of opioids for the management of cancer pain.[16,44] Fear of inducing psychological dependence should never be an indication for withholding appropriate analgesic medication from a child with cancer-related pain.

Additional data to be gathered from patient and family include ascertainment of biases against one or more analgesic strategies or particular drugs. For example, certain families are extremely resistant to the use of any form of invasive procedure, even if medically indicated, in a child with limited life expectancy. Others may refuse morphine because of connotations with drug abuse while hydromorphone or levorphanol may be readily accepted. Although it is generally possible to accommodate such wishes, the health care professional should always remain the advocate for the child's best interest.

The Prior Analgesic History Should Be Reviewed

The most recently used pain control regimens should be reviewed to document the efficacy of any toxicity encountered and to assess the likelihood of physical dependence on opioids, benzodiazepines, or other drugs because abrupt discontinuation of these drugs even after exposures for periods as short as 7–10 days may result in withdrawal symptoms.[45]

The Ability to Tolerate Oral Medication and the Availability of Long-term Venous Access Should Be Assessed

Three further points deserve emphasis. First, the complaint of pain in a child with refractory malignancy should always be believed unless unquestionably proven to be false. Clinical experience indicates that these children, although sometimes apparently exaggerating their degree of suffering, rarely fabricate the actual presence of pain. Second, because it is widely accepted that roughly one-third of patients experiencing documented pain will report some degree of relief from a placebo intervention,[46] the administration of a placebo as a diagnostic test to assess the validity of a child's complaint of pain is scientifically unsound and never clinically indicated. Finally, it should be stressed that appropriate pain management should occur during the evaluation process. The child should not continue in uncontrolled pain during the investigative process.

Therapy Overview

Available analgesic interventions are outlined below. Specific anticancer therapy should be considered even in a child with an apparently very limited life expectancy. This therapy will generally be of a palliative nature, for example, irradiation of painful bone metastases, compressing cord lesions, or intracranial deposits. There are definite indications for the initiation of experimental therapy in children with malignancies refractory to conventional anticancer therapy, provided such therapies are given in a medically sound, legitimate fashion with appropriate informed consent. With this treatment, the child and family are offered the hope of a tumor response, prolongation of life, and decrease in symptomatology. Such therapies must, however, be carefully monitored, and any resulting toxicity managed appropriately.

Irradiation of painful tumor deposits can provide extremely effective pain relief; however, consideration should be given to dose and scheduling details, since daily treatments may place an enormous burden on a sick child. In preterminal children for whom long-term tumor eradication and late effects of irradiation are not an issue, larger fractions can frequently be delivered in a very small number of treatments and provide adequate, albeit temporary, pain relief. The risk-to-benefit ratio should be carefully weighed when irradiation to the abdomen or to mucosal surfaces (e.g., mouth, esophagus, perineum) is being considered since immediate toxicity (nausea, vomiting and diarrhea, and mucosal ulceration, respectively) may be significant.

Surgical intervention for pain relief in the preterminal child is extremely limited but may include procedures such as drainage of a malignant effusion or securing of a drainage pathway from an obstructed, infected organ (e.g., ureteral stent, suprapubic urinary bladder catheter). Bowel obstruction, while once considered an emergent surgical problem, may be amenable to nonsurgical management with analgesics and antispasmodics and decompression with a nasogastric tube and suction. These interventions should be attempted initially before resorting to surgery.

Palliative chemotherapy using conventional agents, as opposed to investigational modalities, may sometimes be highly effective in producing sufficient tumor response to provide pain relief while not producing a documentable partial or complete tumor remission. These palliative chemotherapy regimens should be carefully selected to produce minimal toxicity. An example of palliative chemotherapy is the institution of weekly intravenous vincristine and daily oral prednisone for palliation of refractory acute lymphoblastic leukemia.

Analgesic Interventions

Analgesic interventions include analgesic drugs, anesthetic blocks, inhalational agents, neurosurgical techniques, noninvasive technologies (e.g., TENS, physical therapy), hypnosis, relaxation, and other psychological interventions and supportive and spiritual counseling.

Analgesic Drugs

Administration of analgesic drugs is generally considered to be the primary therapeutic modality for cancer pain relief and for managing the pain of dying children. The major groups of analgesic drugs are nonopioid (aspirin-like) drugs, acetaminophen and nonsteroidal anti-inflammatory agents; opioids, weak and strong; and adjuvant agents. Use of these agents can be considered in two phases: immediate management and chronic management.

> Immediate management of moderate-to-severe pain while evaluating and planning definitive therapy generally requires the administration of a strong opioid drug on a frequent, "as needed," basis to gain initial pain control. This will assure the patient's comfort and his ability to cooperate with necessary evaluation. Chronic management of evaluated, ongoing pain is based on the etiology, nature, and severity of the pain.

The administration of analgesic agents to manage ongoing cancer pain includes a number of important principles.

1. *The administration of a drug should be appropriate to the severity and nature of the pain.* The World Health Organization has developed the

concept of an "analgesic ladder"[47] to guide administration of analgesic drugs to patients with cancer (Figure 2.1). Although nonopioids alone are sufficient to treat mild pain, mild-to-moderate pain requires the use of an opioid drug with or without a nonopioid. A weak opioid such as codeine or oxycodone may be used in initially managing mild-to-moderate or moderate pain; however, some clinicians prefer to begin low dose strong opioid therapy in this situation, particularly if rapid progression of pain is anticipated.[48,49] Should a weak opioid be used, this agent should be discontinued and a strong opioid substituted as soon as progression of pain renders the weak opioid ineffective in producing adequate pain relief. Severe pain always requires the initiation of strong opioid administration. In children, the benefit of adding a nonopioid to a strong opioid regimen has not been adequately studied; however, the use of such a combination may be beneficial. Using adjuvant analgesic drugs should be considered at every step on the ladder.

2. *Regular drug administration to maintain an effective analgesic plasma concentration of drug is optimal.* The administration of regular (immediate-release) oral morphine on a 4 hourly schedule around the clock is an example of this principle. The actual dosing interval for each drug will vary depending on the plasma half-life of the individual drug. Where pain is rapidly escalating, the regularly scheduled drug can be supplemented by additional parenteral or oral opioid doses as needed (PRN) to maintain pain control, and the maintenance dose gradually escalated according to the additional PRN requirement.

3. *Oral drug administration is usually preferable.* Preparation in a flavored liquid vehicle enhances acceptability for many children. In the severely ill, preterminal child, however frequent oral drug administration may be a major burden for the child and caregiver, particularly if this involves awakening the child. When an indwelling intravenous line has

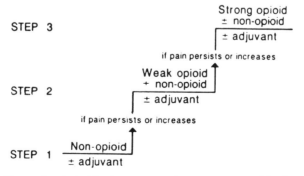

Figure 2.1 The analgesic ladder for cancer pain management. (Freely adapted from Cancer Pain Relief, World Health Organization, 1986.)

been placed, its use for analgesic drug administration may be very effective; however, the major differences in pharmacokinetics following different routes of administration of a single drug should be carefully considered when using this approach.[50] For example, small 3 hourly intravenous morphine boluses may be required to replace 4 hourly oral administration. Such frequent parenteral drug administration may be burdensome to a parent or caregiver. Frequent accessing of an intravenous line also enhances the risk of introducing an infection. More important, intermittent parenteral boluses of an opioid drug may result in "peaks and valleys" of both pain relief and side effects. Ways to avoid this problem include the initiation of a continuous opioid infusion through a pump equipped with a demand bolus option or the use of a "patient controlled analgesia" pump programmed with an appropriate bolus dose and lockout interval permitting bolus administration.[51-55] This pump allows intermittent dosing without repeatedly accessing the intravenous line. A small gauge, indwelling subcutaneous needle placed, for example, in the thoraco-abdominal wall for the purpose of repeated drug administration is another option for patients without long-term intravenous access.[52,56] Needles should be changed every 3–5 days to avoid infection. Complications of this method of drug delivery are uncommon, although local granuloma-like induration has been reported. The use of repeated subcutaneous or intramuscular injections is not an appropriate strategy for children because of the anxiety and pain engendered. Likewise, rectal administration is greatly disliked by children, is not as reliable as other routes since the drugs may be expelled prematurely, and may result in perirectal abscess formation if a mucosal tear results.[57,58] Intranasal and sublingual drug administration have not been studied sufficiently in pediatrics to establish their therapeutic usefulness, although European experience using sublingual buprenorphine is very encouraging.[59]

Finally, transdermal drug administration, using an adhesive patch placed on the skin surface, is a rapidly evolving technology.[60,61] A transdermal therapeutic system containing the strong opioid fentanyl is now approved for use in managing of cancer pain in adults, delivering the equivalent of a constant opioid infusion. The prolonged interval to obtain a steady state plasma concentration of the drug following application of a patch, and the slow decline in the plasma drug concentration following patch removal, makes this methodology currently suitable for relatively stable, ongoing pain rather than the rapidly escalating pain more typical of terminal malignancy in childhood. As methodologies improve, this type of therapy will doubtless become a useful analgesic strategy for pediatrics since no invasive procedures are required.

4. *When a strong opioid is prescribed, individual dosage titration is required* since there is no definable upper dosage limit. Rather, drug doses

should be escalated as required to achieve and maintain adequate pain relief, provided dose-limiting toxicity, particularly respiratory depression, is not encountered. Particularly in the last few days of life, rapid dose escalation is frequently required, demanding careful ongoing evaluation of the child to ensure adequate pain relief.

5. *Adequate sleep at night should be a goal.* Children receiving opioid drugs for management of moderate-to-severe pain frequently lose their regular daytime and nighttime routines, exhibiting instead frequent brief napping during the daytime and prolonged periods of wakefulness at night. Since being awake at night not only is frightening for many children but is also exhausting for family members and caregivers, evening supplementation with a hypnotic agent or antidepressant frequently helps to establish a more normal nighttime sleep pattern.

6. *Side effects of medications should be anticipated* and managed appropriately. For example, the frequent occurrence, but usually transient nature, of opioid-induced somnolence should be discussed with the family when a strong opioid is initially prescribed. Similarly, the almost uniform occurrence of constipation during opioid use should prompt the prescription of a laxative when an opioid drug is begun unless there is an obvious medical contraindication.

7. *The entire medication regime for the dying child should be reviewed* to ensure that only drugs that are absolutely necessary are being prescribed. Taking multiple medications may pose a significant burden and may, in some cases, result in refusal to take vital drugs. Further, such a review will ensure that the potential of drug interactions is addressed prospectively.

8. *The entire analgesic strategy should be discussed with the parents and/or child if appropriate* to ensure their full understanding and to maximize the likelihood of full compliance with the recommended regimen. For example, a family who does not understand the importance of administering analgesics on a regular schedule rather than "as needed" may well wait for breakthrough pain before medicating the child. Further, a family who is suspicious of their child's being overmedicated with a strong opioid may convey this feeling to the child thereby invoking anxiety and guilt in all concerned. An understanding family will be able to provide maximum support for the dying child, to comply with drug administration guidelines, and to reinforce the importance of the analgesic strategy with the child.

Nonopioid "Aspirin-like" Drugs

Acetaminophen is the drug in this category most frequently prescribed in pediatrics. When given in recommended doses (10–12mg/kg orally every 4 hours), it is extremely safe and provides pain relief for mild and mild-to-moderate pain. Aspirin and other nonsteroidal anti-inflammatory drugs are rarely used in managing pediatric cancer pain because they cause gastric irritation that may result in hemorrhage and major disruption of the hemostatic mechanism, particularly by inhibiting platelet function. Further, aspirin use has been associated with the development of Reye's syndrome. Choline salicylate and choline magnesium trisalicylate appear to have little if any effect on gastric mucosa and platelet function and are alternatives to acetaminophen. Their availability in liquid preparation and their efficacy when administered on a 12 hourly schedule makes them potentially useful, albeit poorly studied, for pediatric cancer pain management.

All drugs in this group appear to act peripherally by inhibition of prostaglandin synthesis, and all have anti-inflammatory and antipyretic properties. Although potentially masking of infection-related fever may be of concern for children undergoing intensive chemotherapy with curative intent, this is rarely a clinical issue in the dying patient; indeed, these drugs may provide welcome relief from infection-associated fever.

Weak Opioid Drugs

This group includes the weak opioid agonist drugs and the mixed agonist-antagonist agents. Codeine is the most commonly prescribed $m\mu$ opioid agonist, starting at doses of 0.5mg/kg every 4 hours with escalation to 1–2mg/kg every 4 hours as needed.[48] Unlike strong opioid agents, the weak opioids appear to have a "ceiling effect" of analgesia; escalation beyond the recommended dosage range results in increasing toxicity without a major improvement in pain control. Therefore, if a weak opioid is prescribed but yields inadequate pain relief, its use should be discontinued and a strong opioid instituted. Trials in adults suggest that oxycodone provides excellent pain relief over a broader range of pain, but published data regarding pediatric use is sparse.[48,49] The mixed agonist-antagonist agents have no defined role in managing pediatric cancer pain since they do not appear to provide any benefit when compared with other opioid agents and since they can result in extremely unpleasant dysphoria. The partial $m\mu$ agonist buprenorphine, available for sublingual use in Europe, has been used extensively for pediatric cancer pain relief and appears to have good efficacy and acceptable toxicity.[59] Currently, this drug is only available for parenteral use in the United States.[62]

Strong Opioid Drugs

These drugs are indicated for managing moderate-to-severe pain.[63] Unlike the weak opioid drugs and the nonopioids, there is no definable upper dosage limit for strong opioids. The dose of strong opioids may be escalated as required to achieve and maintain adequate pain relief provided dose-limiting toxicity, particularly respiratory depression, is not encountered.

This results in a very wide interpatient variability in dosage requirements, a phenomenon which should be mentioned to families to avoid the fear that those patients receiving high doses are becoming "addicted." When prescribing strong opioids, it is convenient to consider these agents to be in two categories depending on their plasma half-lives—the short-acting strong opioids with plasma half-lives of 1.5–5 hours, including morphine and hydromorphone, and the longer-acting strong opioids with plasma half-lives of 12–25 hours such as methadone and levorphanol.[64,65]

Morphine, the drug most commonly prescribed, usually orally every 4 hours, rapidly reaches steady state plasma concentrations and can rapidly be titrated to maintain pain relief.[63] Drugs with longer plasma half-lives may require 2–5 days to reach steady state plasma concentrations and are therefore less amenable to rapid changes in dose.[65] If drug escalation of drugs with longer half-lives is performed too quickly, it is possible to experience increasing toxicity over the succeeding 2–4 days as the plasma concentration rises to a steady state. Reflecting this phenomenon are reports in adults of delayed severe respiratory depression during methadone use. The major advantage of a drug with a longer plasma half-life is that it may be administered on a 6 hourly and occasionally 8 hourly schedule thereby decreasing the inconvenience of taking frequent oral medications and permitting undisturbed sleep through much of the night. Sustained-release preparations of morphine are also available, although poorly studied in pediatrics.[66,67] These also offer the possibility of dosing on an 8 or 12 hourly schedule.

With the exception of sustained-release oral morphine preparations, strong opioids are available for both oral and parenteral administration. As stated above, parenteral opioid use is indicated for gaining immediate relief of moderate-to-severe pain, for supplementing analgesia during titration of an oral regimen, and for the child who refuses or is unable to tolerate oral dosing. Many children, who are able to tolerate oral drugs for a prolonged period, require parenteral medications in the preterminal and terminal stages. Because opioid drugs undergo significant first-pass metabolism in the liver following oral administration and because this first-pass effect varies from one drug to another and from one patient to another, converting these agents from oral to parenteral administration should be undertaken only under careful supervision to avoid underdosing or overdosing.[64,68] An example is the oral bioavailability of morphine which, in adults, has been documented to vary between 15–65% and generally, for the purposes of chronic dosing, is averaged to an oral : parenteral dose equivalency of 3 : 1.[64,68] Average conversion ratios are found in Table 2.1; however, the interpatient variability and the effects of organ dysfunction in the indi-

Table 2.1 Nonopioid and Opioid Drugs

Drug	Administration	Comments
Nonopioids		
Acetaminophen	65 mg/kg/day PO; divided doses every 4 hr	These preparations lack gastric ulcerogenic effect and do not inhibit platelet function, common with other non-opioids
Choline magnesium trisalicylate	25 mg/kg every 12 hr PO (adult dose, 1125 mg every 12 hr)	
Weak Opioids		
Codeine	0.5–1 mg/kg PO every 4 hr	Increased toxicity but no increased analgesia with dosages above 1–2 mg/kg PO every 4 hr
Strong Opioids		
Short half-life (1.5–5 hr) Morphine	0.3 mg/kg PO every 4 hr 0.1–0.15 mg/kg IV or IM every 4 hr	Dosage may be escalated to increase analgesic effect
Long half-life (12–25 hr) Methadone	0.6 mg/kg/day PO, divided doses every 4–6 hr 0.3–0.45 mg/kg/day IV or IM, divided doses every 4–6 hr	Dosage may be escalated to increase analgesic effect; accumulation may occur, resulting in delayed respiratory depression
Sustained-release morphine preparations	0.9 mg/kg every 12 hr PO 0.6 mg/kg every 8 hr PO	Dosage titration required

Modified from Pizzo P, Poplack D. Principles and Practice of Pediatric Oncology, Philadelphia, J. B. Lippincott, 1989, page 927; with permission.

vidual child should be taken into consideration when such a conversion is considered.

The toxicity encountered during strong opioid use is outlined in Table 2.2. Although all agents carry the same range of potential toxicity, an individual child may experience toxicity with one strong opioid but not another. For example, nausea and vomiting experienced with morphine may be avoided by a change to hydromorphone or methadone. Constipation is almost always seen with all narcotic analgesics and should be managed prophylactically. Initial somnolence is usually transient; persistent somnolence may occasionally be managed by a psychostimulant drug such as methylphenidate, although its efficacy in pediatrics is purely anecdotal. Severe, persistent drowsiness should prompt consideration of other analgesic strategies such as local nerve block or epidural infusions as discussed in

Table 2.2 Opioid Side Effects

Side Effect	Management
Respiratory depression	Reduction in opioid dose
Respiratory arrest	Naloxone 0.01–0.1 mg/kg IV or IM; rarely indicated in terminally ill child (see text)
	Small frequent doses of diluted naloxone or naloxone drip preferable for patients on chronic opioid therapy to avoid severe, painful withdrawal syndrome. Repeated doses often required until opioid effect subsides. Intubation may be required because naloxone frequently induces vomiting
Drowsiness/sedation	Frequently subsides after a few days without dosage reduction; methylphenidate or dexto-amphetamine may be useful in adults (inadequate pediatric data)
Constipation	Prophylactic laxatives indicated
Nausea/vomiting	Change to a different narcotic may alleviate symptoms; hydroxyzine or a phenothiazine drug often beneficial but may cause increased sedation
Euphoria, confusion, nightmares, hallucinations	Reassurance only, if symptoms mild; change to a different opioid may avoid symptoms. Haloperidol may be beneficial
Multifocal myoclonus; seizures	Generally occur only during extremely high-dose therapy; reduction in opioid dose indicated if possible
Urinary retention	Rule out bladder outlet obstruction, neurogenic bladder and other precipitating drugs (e.g., tricyclic antidepressant). Particulary common with epidural opioids. Change of opioid, route of administration, and dose may relieve symptom. Bethanechol, crede, or catheter may be required
Allergic Phenomena	
Urticaria	Change to opioid of different structure (e.g., morphine to methadone) required
Itching	Antihistamine (e.g., hydroxyzine) often beneficial
Related Manifestations	
Tolerance	Escalate drug dosage as required. If clinically problematic, change to a different drug or route of administration may be indicated
Physical dependence	Taper drug doses slowly to avoid withdrawal symptoms
Psychological dependence ("addiction")	Rarely induced by therapeutic use of opioids in cancer patients

Modified from Pizzo P, Poplack D. Principles and Practice of Pediatric Oncology, Philadelphia, J.B. Lippincott, 1989, page 928; with permission.

the section "Other Analgesic Approaches." The most important potential complication is respiratory depression. Respiratory rates of 12 breaths per minute and above require no intervention. Respiratory rates below 12 per minute may require a decrease in the opioid dose, although the terminally ill child displaying 8–10 breaths per minute while asleep and enjoying good pain relief usually requires no intervention. For major respiratory depression, the use of an opioid antagonist such as naloxone requires extremely careful forethought and consideration before administration since an extremely unpleasant and excruciatingly painful withdrawal syndrome may be precipitated. Vomiting with the potential for aspiration may also occur. In the rare cases when naloxone is indicated, extremely dilute solutions should be used and administered intravenously as a slow injection to reestablish breathing yet avoid withdrawal. Other side effects may be managed by either symptomatic measures or by a trial of switching from one strong opioid to another. Examples of symptomatic management include administering of antihistamines for itching and using antiemetics for nausea and vomiting. Nightmares and occasional hallucinations appear to occur frequently in pediatrics particularly in the preterminal child. These rarely require specific management, although small doses of haloperidol may decrease this symptom. Large doses of phenothiazine for any indication should be avoided since children display a high incidence of extrapyramidal reactions, particularly dystonia, during use of these drugs. A final note of caution is that, during high dose parenteral morphine administration, a preservative-free preparation should be used since morphine solutions containing the preservative chlorbutanol have been associated with extreme somnolence.

It should be noted that meperidine has been excluded from the above discussion since repeated use, particularly in patients with renal compromise, has been associated with central nervous system excitability and convulsions due to the accumulation of the toxic metabolite normeperidine. Since this drug has no analgesic benefit when compared with other strong opioids, its use in managing pediatric cancer pain should be restricted to the occasional child who develops side effects with other strong opioids but is able to tolerate meperidine and experiences good pain relief.

Other Analgesic Approaches

Other analgesic approaches include adjuvant use of other nonanalgesic drugs, anesthetic nerve blocks, noninvasive techniques, and neurosurgical approaches. The use of adjuvant drugs is discussed in the following section and in the "Symptom Control" section earlier. Anesthetic nerve blocks, although used in adult cancer patients, are rarely indicated in children because of the widespread nature of most terminal childhood malignancies.

Peripheral nerve blocks on the trunk, where interruption of both motor and sensory components will not pose a functional problem,[69] autonomic nerve blocks, celiac plexus nerve block[70] (for refractory upper abdominal pain), and epidural nerve blocks[71] (for abdominal, lumbosacral, sacral, and perineal pain) can be considered for specific pain syndromes. Unless the dying child already knows hypnosis, a relaxation technique, these modalities cannot be easily taught in the terminal days of life. Very rarely, neurosurgical spinal cord ablation is necessary for extremely severe pain uncontrolled by high dose intravenous narcotics.

Adjuvant Drugs

These drugs are not primarily analgesic. Nevertheless, while being developed to treat other symptoms, it was incidentally found that they produce analgesia under some circumstances.[72,73] Glucocorticosteroids have been found to be effective in treating bone pain caused by tumor invading bone typically seen in neuroblastoma, Ewing's sarcoma, and leukemia. As discussed in an earlier section, anticonvulsants and antidepressants are often effective in treating neuropathic pain.

THE DEATH PROCESS

A gradual and peaceful death process can usually be achieved. The emotional, physical, and spiritual environments for the child's death are generally carefully determined by the child and the family with the help of the hospice team. A quiet, comfortable, peaceful, clean, ordered, private room is usually optimal. This environment will allow those with special relationships to share an important time together. The hospice team can play a very important role in controlling the acute symptoms during the final death process. This will allow the final hours of life to be meaningful without objectionable, disruptive, and uncomfortable symptoms that are difficult for the dying child and those around him or her. Complete control of pain is of utmost importance. The dose of narcotic may need to be increased significantly in the last few hours of life to avoid discomfort. Thus, monitoring of pain control by the hospice team should be intensified to assure a rapid response to changes in pain.

The terminal process is usually manifested by a gradual decline in the respiratory effort and effective ventilation resulting in hypoxia and a rise in carbon dioxide. If there is significant pulmonary pathology, for example, pulmonary edema, ventilation-perfusion inequalities may occur resulting in more significant hypoxia. Hypoxia results in agitation while hypercarbia results in somnolence; thus, treating hypoxia aggressively with oxygen is essential to a peaceful death. The agitation of hypoxia may be difficult to distinguish from pain because agitation may be the only way for the child to communicate distress; however, the treatment of both causes of agitation is adequate narcotic therapy.[4] Adequate control of terminal agitation is usually best effected by a continuous infusion of narcotics. Using this method of administration, the dose can be easily adjusted without bolus effects on the level of consciousness and respiratory drive and without any peaks and valleys of analgesic effect. Additional sedation with thorazine or haloperidol may also be beneficial. Muscle twitching may require the addition of a benzodiazepine: lorazepam (Ativan) or diazepam (Valium).[4] Terminal seizures may occasionally be seen. If they occur they must be anticipated and treated quickly with anticonvulsants to avoid emotional distress for the family, friends, and child.

As the child becomes weaker, he or she may become too weak to clear his or her airway secretions. This results in noisy breath sounds that may cause distress for the family and friends. The hospice team can play an important role in allaying the fear that the child is suffering or in distress because of this. Scopolamine given subcutaneously may help considerably in drying up excessive secretions while relaxing the smooth muscle of the tracheobronchial tree.

In summary, in order for a peaceful death process to occur, each symptom must be meticulously anticipated and treated. Successful prevention and treatment of symptoms allows the quiet completion of relationships between the dying child and those significant people in his or her life.

NOTES

1. Walsh TD, Saunders CM: Hospice care: The treatment of pain in advanced cancer. Recent Results Cancer Res 89:201–211, 1984.

2. Norton WS, Lack SA: Control of symptoms other than pain, in Twycross RG, Ventafridda V (eds): The Continuing Care of Terminal Cancer Patients. Oxford, Pergamon Press, p 167, 1980.

3. Doyle D: Palliative symptom control, in Doyle D (ed): Palliative Care: The Management of Far Advanced Illness. Philadelphia, Charles Press, p 297, 1984.

4. Levy MH, Catalano RB: Control of common physical symptoms other than pain in patients with terminal disease. Sem in Oncol 12:411–430, 1985.

5. Cunningham D, Turner A, Hawthorn J, Rosin RD: Ondansetron with and without dexamethasone to treat chemotherapy-induced emesis. Lancet 1: 1323, 1989.

6. Sagar SM: The current role of anti-emetic drugs in oncology: A recent revolution in patient symptom control. Cancer Treat Rev 18:95–135, 1991.

7. Laszlo J, Clark RA, Hanson DC, Tyson L, Crumpler L, Gralla R: Lorazepam in cancer patients treated with cisplatin: a drug having antiemetic, amnesic, and anxiolytic effects. J Clin Oncol 3:864–869, 1985.

8. Frytak S, Moertel CG: Management of nausea and vomiting in the cancer patient. JAMA 245:393–396, 1981.

9. Cassileth PA, Lusk EJ, Torri S, DiNubile N, Gerson SL: Antiemetic efficacy of dexamethasone therapy in patients receiving cancer chemotherapy. Arch Intern Med 143:1347–1349, 1983.

10. Coyle JR: The clinical role of antipsychotic medications. Med Clin North Am 66:993–1010, 1982.

11. Rosenbaum JF: The drug treatment of anxiety. N Engl J Med 306:401–404, 1982.

12. Woodcock AA, Gross ER, Gellert AG, et al: Effects of dihydrocodeine, alcohol, and caffeine on breathlessness and exercise tolerance in patients with chronic obstructive lung disease and normal blood gases. N Engl J Med 305:1611–1616, 1981.

13. Klein H: Constipation and fecal impaction. Med Clin North Am 66:1135–1142, 1982.

14. Foltz AT: Nursing care of ulcerating metastatic lesions. Oncol Nurs Forum 7:8–13, 1980.

15. Reuler JB, Cooney TG: The pressure sore: Pathophysiology and principles of management. Ann Intern Med 94:661–666, 1981.

16. Miser AW, Dothage JA, Wesley RA, et al: The prevalence of pain in a pediatric and young adult cancer population. Pain 29:73–83, 1987.

17. Daut RL, Cleeland CS: The prevalence and severity of pain in cancer. Cancer 50:1913–1918, 1982.

18. Oster MW, Vizel M, Turgeon LR: Pain of terminal cancer patients. Arch Intern Med 138:1801–1802, 1978.

19. Coyle N, Adelhardt J, Foley KM, Portenoy RK. Character of terminal illness in the advanced cancer patient. Pain and other symptoms during the last four weeks of life. J Pain Symptom Manage 5:83–93, 1990.

20. McGrath PJ, Hsu E, Cappelli M, Luke B, Goodman JT, Dunn-Geier J. Pain from pediatric cancer: A survey of an outpatient oncology clinic. J Psychosoc Oncol 8:109–124, 1990.

21. Coyle N, Adelhardt J, Foley KM, Portenoy RK. Character of terminal illness in the advanced cancer patient: Pain and other symptoms during the last four weeks of life. J Pain Symptom Manage 5:83–93, 1990.

22. Maunuksela EL, Saatiner UM, Lahteenoja KM. Relevance and management of terminal pain in children with cancer: Five-year experience in Helsinki, Finland. Adv Pain Res Ther 15:383–390, 1990.

23. Procacci P, Maresca M. Reflex sympathetic dystrophies and algodystrophies: historical and pathogenic considerations. Pain 31:137–146, 1987.

24. Greipp ME, Thomas AF, Renkun C. Children and young adults with reflex sympathetic dystrophy syndrome. Clin J Pain 4:217–221, 1988.

25. Savedra M, Gibbons P, Tesler M, et al: How do children describe pain? A tentative assessment. Pain 14:95–104, 1982.

26. Gaffney A. How children describe pain: A study of words and analogies used by 5–14-year-olds. In Dubner R, Gebhardt G, Bond M (eds): Pain Research and Clinical Management, vol. 3. Amsterdam, Elsevier, 1988, pp. 341–347.

27. Melzack R. The McGill pain questionnaire: Major properties and scoring methods. Pain 1:277–299, 1975.

28. Katz ER, Varni JW, Jay SM: Behavioral assessment and management of pediatric pain. Prog Behav Modif 18:163–193, 1984.

29. Dothage JA, Arndt C, Miser AW: Use of a continuous intravenous morphine infusion for pain control in an infant with terminal malignancy. J Assoc Pediatr Oncol Nurs 3:22–24, 1986.

30. McGrath PJ, Beyer J, Cleeland C, Eland J, McGrath PA, Portenoy R. Report of the subcommittee on assessment and methodologic issues in the management of pain in childhood cancer. Pediatr 86:814–817, 1990.

31. McGrath PJ, Johnson GR, Goodman JT, et al: The development and validation of a behavioral pain scale for children: The Children's Hospital of Eastern Ontario Pain Scale (CHEOPS). Pain (Suppl 2):S24, 1984.

32. Teske K, Daut RL, Cleeland CS: Relationships between nurses' observations and patients' self-reports of pain. Pain 16:289–296, 1983.

33. Gauvain-Piquard A, Rodary C, Rezvani A, Lemerle J: Pain in children aged 2–6 years: A new observational rating scale elaborated in a pediatric oncology unit. Preliminary report. Pain 31:177–188, 1987.

34. Lollar DJ, Smits SJ, Patterson DL: Assessment of pediatric pain: An empirical perspective. J Pediatr Psychol 7:267–277, 1982.

35. Beyer J: The Ocuher: A User's Manual and Technical Report. Denver, Colorado, University of Colorado Health Sciences Center, 1988.

36. Pothmann J, Goepel R: Comparison of the visual analog scale (VAS) and the Smiley analog scale (SAS) for the evaluation of pain in children. Pain (Suppl 2):S25, 1984.

37. Gracely RH: Psychophysical assessment of human pain. Adv Pain Res Ther 3:805–824, 1979.

38. Szyfelbein SK, Osgood PF, Carr DB: The assessment of pain and plasma beta-endorphin immunoreactivity in burned children. Pain 22:173–182, 1985.

39. Eland JM: The child who is hurting. Semin Oncol Nurs 1:116–122, 1985.

40. Hester NK: The preoperational child's perspective to immunization. Nurs Res 28:250–255, 1979.

41. LeBaron S, Zeltzer L: Assessment of acute pain and anxiety in children and adolescents by self reports, observer reports, and a behavioral checklist. J Consult Clin Psychol 52:729–738, 1984.

42. Elliott SC, Miser AW, Dose AM, et al: Epidemiologic features of pain in pediatric cancer patients. A cooperative community-based study. Clin J Pain 7:263–268, 1991.

43. Jaffe JH: Drug addiction and drug abuse. In Gilman AG, Goodman LS, Gilman A (eds): The Pharmacological Basis of Therapeutics, 6th ed, pp 535–584, New York, Macmillan, 1980.

44. Kanner RM, Foley KM: Patterns of narcotic drug use in a cancer pain clinic. Ann NY Acad Sci 362, 161–172, 1981.

45. Miser AW, Chayt KJ, Sandlund JT, et al: Narcotic withdrawal syndrome in young adults after the therapeutic use of opiates. Am J Dis Child 140:603–604, 1986.

46. Levine JD, Gordon NC: Influence of the method of drug administration on analgesic response. Nature 312:755–766, 1984.

47. World Health Organization: Cancer Pain Relief. Geneva, World Health Organization, 1986.

48. Beaver WT, Wallenstein SL, Rogers A, Houde RW: Analgesic studies of codeine and oxycodone in patients with cancer. I. Comparison of oral with intramuscular codeine and of oral intramuscular oxycodone. J Pharm Exp Ther 207:92–100, 1978.

49. Kalso E, Vainio A: Morphine and oxycodone hydrochloride in the management of cancer pain. Clin Pharmacol Ther 47:639–645, 1990.

50. Lacouture PG, Gauderault P, Lovejoy FH: Chronic pain of childhood: A pharmacological approach. Pediatr Clin North Am 31:1133–1151, 1984.

51. Miser AW, Miser JS, Clark BW: Continuous intravenous infusion of morphine sulfate for control of severe pain in children with terminal malignancy. J Pediatr 96:930–932, 1980.

52. Miser AW, Moore L, Greene R, et al: Prospective study of continuous intravenous and subcutaneous morphine infusions for therapy-related or cancer-related pain in children and young adults with cancer. Clin J Pain 2:101–106, 1986.

53. Baumann TJ, Batenhorst RL, Graves DA, et al: Patient-controlled analgesia in the terminally ill cancer patient. Drug Intell Clin Pharm 20:297–301, 1986.

54. Tyler DC: Patient controlled analgesia in adolescents. J Adolesc Health Care 11:154–158, 1990.

55. Berde C, Lehn BM, Yee JD, Sethna NF, Russo D: Patient-controlled analgesia in children and adolescents: A randomized, prospective comparison with intramuscular administration of morphine for postoperative analgesia. J Pediatr 118: 460–466, 1991.

56. Miser AW, Davis DM, Hughes CS, et al: Continuous subcutaneous infusion of morphine in children in cancer. Am J Dis Child 137:383–385, 1983.

57. Ellison NM, Lewis GO: A pharmacokinetic comparison of rectal morphine sulfate (RMS) suppositories and oral morphine sulfate (OMS) solution. Proc Am Soc Clin Oncol 3:89, 1984.

58. Brook-Williams P, Hoover LH: Morphine suppositories for intractable pain. Can Med Assoc J 126:14, 1982.

59. Massimo L, Haupt R, Zamorani ME: Control of pain with sublingual buprenorphine in children with cancer. Eur Paediatr Haematol Oncol 2:224, 1985.

60. Miser AW, Narang PK, Dothage JA, et al: Transdermal fentanyl for pain control in patients with cancer. Pain 37:15–21, 1989.

61. Simmonds MA, Payne R, Richenbacher J, et al: TTS (fentanyl) in the management of pain in patients with cancer. Proc Ann Meet Am Soc Clin Oncol 8:PA 1260, 1989.

62. Maunuksela EL, Korpela R, Ilkkola KT: Comparison of buprenorphine with morphine in the treatment of postoperative pain in children. Anesth Analg 67:233–239, 1988.

63. Walsh TD: Oral morphine in chronic cancer pain. Pain 18:1–11, 1984.

64. Neumann PB, Henriksen H, Grosman N, et al: Plasma morphine concentrations during chronic oral administration in patients with cancer pain. Pain 13:247–252, 1982.

65. Nilsson MI, Meresaar U, Anggard E: Clinical pharmacokinetics of methadone. Acta Anaesth Scan Suppl 74:66–69, 1982.

66. Homesley HD, Welander CE, Muss HB, et al: Dosage range study of morphine sulfate controlled-release. Am J Clin Oncol 9:449–453, 1986.

67. Warfield C: Evaluation of dosing guidelines for the use of oral controlled-release morphine (MS Contin tablets). Cancer 63:2360–2364, 1989.

68. Nahata MC, Miser AW, Miser JS, et al: Variations in morphine pharmacokinetics in children with cancer. Dev Pharmacol Ther 8:182–188, 1986.

69. Dalens B: Regional anesthesia in children. Anesth Analg 68:654–672, 1989.

70. Berde CB, Sethna NF, Fisher DE, Kahn CH, Chandler P, Grier HE: Celiac

plexus blockade for a 3-year-old boy with hepatoblastoma and refractory pain. Pediatrics 86:779–781, 1990.

71. Cousin MJ, Bridenbaugh PO (eds): Neural Blockade in Clinical Anesthesia and the Management of Pain. Philadelphia, JB Lippincott, 1980.

72. Rosenblatt RM, Reich J, Dehring D: Tricyclic antidepressants in treatment of depression and chronic pain: Analysis of the supporting evidence. Anesth Analg 63:1025–1032, 1984.

73. Swerdlow M: Anticonvulsant drugs and chronic pain. Clin Neuropharm 7: 51–82, 1984.

SUGGESTED READINGS ON PAIN

Cancer Pain Relief. Geneva, World Health Organization, 1986.

Doyle D. Palliative symptom control. In Doyle D (ed). Palliative Care: The Management of Far Advanced Illness. Philadelphia, Charles Press, 1984.

Greene MG (ed). The Harriet Lane Handbook. St. Louis, Mosby-Year Book, 1991.

Levy MH, Catalano RB. Control of common physical symptoms other than pain in patients with terminal disease. Sem in Oncology 12:411–430, 1985.

Miser AW, Miser JS, Clark BW. Continuous infusion of morphine sulfate for control of severe pain in children with terminal malignancy. J Pediatr 96:930–932, 1980.

Norton ES, Lack SA. Control of symptoms other than pain. In Twycross RG, Ventafridda V (eds). The Continuing Care of Terminal Cancer Patients. Oxford, Pergamon Press, 1980.

Pizzo P, Poplack D (eds). Principles and Practice of Pediatric Oncology, Philadelphia, J.B. Lippincott, 1989.

3

Psychosocial Aspects of Serious Illness in Childhood and Adolescence

MARTHA BLECHAR GIBBONS

Life-threatening, chronic illnesses affecting children cause chaos within the family system and disruption of the family equilibrium. Families find themselves challenged by multiple, powerful stresses, related to the medical diagnosis, the treatment, the course of the disease, and the possible fatal outcome. Although initial shock, anger, and chaos occur at the time of diagnosis, family members experience continuous fear, disbelief, anxiety, pain, stress, and feelings of being on an "emotional roller coaster."

Serious illness affects children of different ages in many ways. It creates the threat of the unknown, loss of control, additional tasks for children to master, and long-term effects.

Petrillo and Sanger[1] describe eleven concerns for the ill child who requires hospitalization: an imperfect body; the degree of illness requiring hospitalization; threatened or real hospitalization; spending time with unfamiliar people; difficulty maintaining contact with siblings and peers; possible painful procedures; feelings of guilt toward self or parents for hospitalization; unfamiliar routines and environment; placement of parents in a helpless role; the need for the child to be in a dependent role; and the need to relate to health professionals who may appear frightening.

IMPACT OF ILLNESS ON THE INFANT

In infancy, the developmental task is to achieve an awareness of being separate from a significant other.[2] Serious illness in the first year of life can alter the development of self-awareness. Treatment may result in separation from the mother, pain due to invasive procedures, and forced alterations in diet and sleeping habits. The infant's inability to comprehend the disease cognitively contributes to the parents' despair because they are unable to offer explanations and reassurance to the child. Psychologic and emotional trauma related to the disease may distort the normal processes of differentiation of self from mother.

Infants learn primarily through motor activity that may be goal oriented or through impulsive tension release. In supporting the infant who is experiencing serious illness, it is important to be sensitive to a need to engage in body rocking, toy manipulation, and crying, and to bring attention to those needs.

Whenever possible, parents should be encouraged to remain with their infant, to bathe the infant, and to talk with the child. When they have to be absent, parents can be encouraged to tape their voices (reading, singing) and have the tapes played by those attending the infant.

The provision of visual and auditory stimulation is essential, even for the critically ill child. Mobiles with a visible surface (i.e., flat underneath) in bright colors or black and white contrasts are recommended. Music should be calming and, if possible, familiar to the child. The crib or nursery area should be maintained as a safe and calming place, where no invasive procedures are performed. (See Table 3.1.)

IMPACT OF ILLNESS ON THE TODDLER

For the toddler, the major developmental task is initiating the evolution of autonomy or self-control,[2] outcomes that are jeopardized when the small child becomes seriously ill. The toddler's egocentrism, lack of concept of infinite time, and inability to distinguish between fact and fantasy prevent comprehension of the concept of death. Death at this stage of development may mean separation from what the child holds dear.

The most frightening aspects of illness and hospitalization for the toddler usually include pain, anxiety, and separation from parents, but not anxiety about death. The oedipal-age child is especially sensitive to bodily harm and may be particularly traumatized by invasive procedures. The dying toddler will respond with fear or sadness to the anxiety, sadness, fear, depression, or anger expressed by parents and other significant others, rather than the fear of death.

The most common and most effective coping method employed by the seriously ill toddler is regression. Regression may be physiologic, as when a toddler refuses to continue bowel or bladder training, or emotional, as when a child who was verbal refuses to talk, withdraws, or becomes easily irritated and angry. Regression involves the loss of newly acquired achievements and may be frightening to the toddler.

Parents may be reluctant to enforce discipline with the seriously ill child because of their guilt feelings and realistic concern regarding the child's

Table 3.1   The Illness Experience: The Child and Adolescent

Infant

Developmental Task   Achievement of awareness of being separate from significant other
Impact of Illness   Potential distortion of differentiation of self from parent/significant others
Cognitive Age/Stage   Sensorimotor (birth through 2 years)
Major Fears   Separation, strangers
Interventions   Provide consistent caretakers. Minimize separation from parents/significant others. Decrease parental anxiety, which is projected to infant. Maintain crib/nursery as "safe place" where no invasive procedures are performed.

Toddler

Developmental Task   Initiation of autonomy
Impact of Illness   Interference with/loss of developing sense of control, independence
Cognitive Age/Stage   Preoperational thought (2–7 years): egocentric, magical, little concept of body integrity
Major Fears   Separation, loss of control
Concept of Illness   Phenomenism (2–7 years): Perceives external, unrelated, concrete phenomena as cause of illness, e.g., "being sick because you don't feel well." Contagion: Perceives cause of illness as proximity between two events that occurs by "magic," e.g., "getting a cold because you are near someone who has a cold."
Interventions   Minimize separation from parents/significant others. Keep security objects at hand. Provide simple, brief explanations. Explain and maintain consistent limits. Encourage participation in daily care, etc. Provide opportunities for play/play therapy.

Preschooler

Developmental Task   Creation of a sense of initiative
Impact of Illness   Interference/loss of accomplishments such as walking, talking, controlling basic bodily functions
Cognitive Age/Stage   Preoperational thought: egocentric, magical, tendency to use and repeat words they don't understand, providing own explanations and definitions. Literal translation of words. Inability to abstract.
Major Fears   Bodily injury and mutilation; loss of control; the unknown; the dark; being left alone.
Concept of Illness   Phenomenism; Contagion.
Interventions   Provide simple, concrete explanations. Advance preparation is important: days for major events, hours for minor events. Verbal explanations are usually insufficient, so use pictures, models, actual equipment, medical play.

(continued)

---

condition. The child may overreact emotionally to inconsistency in discipline patterns. Without consistent limitations, the toddler feels insecure and is unable to complete developmental tasks essential to the promotion of autonomy. Parents should be encouraged to maintain the child's normal schedule as much as possible and to explain and maintain consistent limits.

IMPACT OF ILLNESS ON THE PRESCHOOLER

The chief developmental task of the preschooler is to create a sense of initiative. Important accomplishments include walking, talking, controlling basic bodily functions, and being separate from the mother.[2]

Table 3.1   *Continued*

School-Age Child

Developmental Task   Development of a sense of industry

Impact of Illness   Potential feelings of inadequacy/inferiority if autonomy and independence are compromised.

Cognitive Age/Stage   Concrete operational thought (7–10+ years): beginning of logical thought but tendency to be literal.

Major Fears   Loss of control; bodily injury and mutilation; failure to live up to expectations of important others; death.

Concept of Illness   Contamination: Perceives cause as a person, object, or action external to the child that is "bad" or "harmful" to the body, e.g., "getting a cold because you didn't wear a hat." Internalization: Perceives illness as having an external cause but being located inside the body, e.g., "getting a cold by breathing in air and bacteria."

Interventions   Provide choices whenever possible to increase the child's sense of control. Stress contact with peer group. Use diagrams, pictures, and models for explanations because thinking is concrete. Emphasize the "normal" things the child can do, since the child does not want to be seen as different. Reassure child he/she has done nothing wrong; hospitalization, etc. is not "punishment."

Adolescent

Developmental Task   Achievement of a sense of identity

Impact of Illness   Potential alteration/relinquishment of newly acquired roles and responsibilities

Cognitive Age/Stage   Formal operational thought (11+ years): beginning of ability to think abstractly. Existence of some magical thinking (e.g., feeling guilty for illness) and egocentrism

Major Fears   Loss of control; altered body image; separation from peer group

Concept of Illness   Physiologic: Perceives cause as malfunctioning or nonfunctioning organ or process; can explain illness in sequence of events. Psychophysiologic: Realizes that psychologic actions and attitudes affect health and illness.

Interventions   Allow adolescent to be an integral part of decision making regarding care. Give information sensitively, since this age group reacts to content of information as well as the manner in which it is delivered. Allow as many choices and as much control as possible. Be honest about treatment and consequences. Stress what the adolescent can do for him or herself and the importance of cooperation and compliance. Assist in maintaining contact with peer group.

Source: Data on concept of illness for table obtained from Bibace, R, & Walsh, ME: Development of children's concepts of illness. Pediatrics 66:912–918, 1980.

The preschooler's conscience is uncompromising. Thoughts about "bad things" or wishing for "bad things" to happen to others lead to feelings of guilt and anxiety. Painful treatments, isolation, separation from parents, loss of autonomy, and immobilization are likely to be interpreted as punishment for real or imagined wrongdoing.

The preschooler may react aggressively to the impact of illness and disease by throwing toys, biting, and hitting others. The preschooler may regress, withdraw from others, wet the bed, have difficulty sleeping, or refuse to cooperate.

Young children accept the literal meaning of words. If death has been associated with "going to sleep" in an explanation, the child may fear going to sleep and never waking up. The child may be plagued by nightmares symbolizing illness-related fears. It is important to provide the opportunity for the child to express those fears and frustrations. At this age, the use of storytelling or books that address the topic of illness and death indirectly (such as in stories about animals or nature) may be beneficial in providing a nonthreatening approach to this topic. Children often are more able to express concerns in dramatic play.

At this age, a sense of security is derived from schedules and rules. Parents should be encouraged to maintain the normal schedule and consistent limits, whenever possible.

One of the defense mechanisms used most commonly by young children to deal with loss is denial. Fewer defense mechanisms are available to a child of this age for dealing with issues related to death and dying.

A child of this age needs constant reassurance that nothing he or she has done has caused the illness; that it is not a form of punishment. Honesty is important, as are explanations regarding deviations from routines or changes in plans. Because the child has a very limited concept of time, attaching explanations to known events (e.g., "after your nap" or "after lunch") helps to avoid confusion.

IMPACT OF ILLNESS ON THE SCHOOL-AGE CHILD

During the school-age period, the child has achieved a certain degree of autonomy and independence and strives to develop a sense of industry. The child is capable of higher thought processes. Use of concrete operations is also characteristic of this age.[2]

The school-age child takes pride in the ability to assume new responsibilities; with increasing independence comes increasing self-esteem. If the child experiences repeated failures or frustrations in attempts at achievement during this period, however, a sense of inadequacy or inferiority may develop instead.

Peer relationships and peer approval become increasingly important at this age. Separation from the peer group is often a significant and difficult consequence of illness. Whenever possible, it is beneficial for the child to maintain contact with friends.

Children at this age have the ability to listen attentively to all that is said but without always comprehending. Therefore, to avoid misconceptions, it is most helpful to ask the child to explain what he or she knows or understands. There is a reluctance at this age to ask questions or admit not knowing something they think they are expected to know.

The school-age child has an increased awareness of the significance of various illnesses, the potential hazards of treatments, the lifelong consequences of injury, and the concept of death. It is important to anticipate and answer questions regarding the long-term consequences of treatments, for example, what the scar will look like after surgery. Reassurance is still needed that the child has done nothing to cause his or her illness.

Terminally ill school-age children are often aware of their fatal prognosis without being told. They are acutely aware of nonverbal clues and often understand much more than their parents or caregivers realize. For this reason, it is important to encourage those caring for the child to maintain open, honest communication. Open communication allows the child an opportunity to discuss fears and apprehensions and therefore not bear the burden erroneous assumptions might yield. The child can then be assisted to work through fears and to find more effective coping strategies.

Unstructured play remains an important aspect of the school-aged child's life. It enhances the child's feelings of control and predictability. Play also serves both as a temporary escape from the stresses of seriousness illness and as a vehicle for resolving emotions. It is important to provide age-appropriate materials for the child. It may be necessary to play for those children who are physically or emotionally unable to engage in play, involving the child to whatever extent is possible.

IMPACT OF ILLNESS ON THE ADOLESCENT

For the adolescent, the diagnosis of a life-threatening illness comes at a time when questions such as "Who am I?" and "What am I about?" are being posed. Adolescence is a time of increasing independence, autonomy, and vulnerability. It is a time in life when self-esteem is closely linked with peer acceptance. Adolescents come to accept and like who they are partly as a result of being accepted and supported by their peers.[2] The adolescent's need to be in harmony with peers in all aspects of appearance and life-style make drug side effects such as weight gain, acne, and hair loss particularly troublesome. All these changes may have a negative impact on the adolescent's self esteem.[3]

All too often "adolescence" is considered one stage, rather than three distinct stages of development each with its own unique characteristics. An adolescent of 11 experiences things much differently than an adolescent of 19. To complicate matters, adolescents may be placed in pediatric wards in some institutions, and in others, included in adult units and treated as "adults."

Early adolescence (approximately ages 11–13 for girls, 12–14 for boys) marks the beginning of puberty, when the body starts to change overtly. There is an increased awareness of sexuality, and the first erotic sexual feelings are experienced, along with increased feelings of awkwardness with the opposite gender. This time also marks the beginning of authority challenges. Peers during this time become as important as parents (a change that is manifested by increasing parent-child conflicts). There are volatile friendships; the loss of a friend is significant at this age. Early adolescence is an emotionally vulnerable period because of the hormonal influences, the sense of loss of childhood, and the anxiety experienced in relation to all the other changes taking place. There is "magical thinking" at this age, and consequences of behaviors are considered in a fairly remote manner. "The future" is fairly close (such as the dance in a few months). The child in this age is still concrete in his or her thinking.

Middle adolescence (approximately ages 14–15 for girls, 15–17 for boys) marks "more of everything" that occurred earlier: there is more challenging of authority figures, more questioning of parental values, and an upsurge in cognitive skills. Adolescents at this age rarely consider the consequences of their behaviors. The present is most important, although there is the capacity to look toward the future. The sense of invulnerability is strong at this stage of development, and risk-taking behavior is more frequent. This sense of immortality makes it especially difficult to deal with issues regarding death and loss. Peers are more important than ever, which makes group support and peer education more favorable supportive interventions. There is a strong sense of inadequacy, and often the adolescent holds on to a relationship for a sense of "grounding."

Late adolescence (approximately ages 16–19 for girls, 17–19 for boys) marks the period in which the individual becomes more future-oriented. Now the adolescent is capable of thinking of the future (such as retirement) and possesses a fully developed abstract thinking process. Feelings of inadequacy now are more reality-based because this age is closer to the experience. The individual now appreciates more the meaning of loss ("I'll never be able to play basketball professionally") more than he or she could at an earlier stage of development. For many, there is an increasing sense of competency with the development of skills. Parents during this period "reemerge" in importance, as the individual gravitates back to appreciate family values.

During adolescence, both sexes are developing their sexual identity. Certain changes, such as hair loss, may be experienced by adolescents as devastating to their self-image. Loss of hair may signify a loss of beauty to girls and a loss of masculinity to boys.[4]

The diagnosis and treatment of a life-threatening illness forces the adolescent to relinquish or alter some of the roles that he or she has previously assumed and to take on at least one new role—that of patient.

Adolescents are emerging from the relative dependency of childhood and are trying to establish their independence outside the family. However, they still have strong needs for nurturance, acceptance, and direction from their parents, which often creates conflict and upsets the balance between what the adolescent needs and what they will accept. Adolescents faced with a chronic illness must learn to accept help from others where previously they were able to function independently. For some, the side effects of the treatment or the debilitating nature of the disease itself will inhibit meeting even the most basic needs. Dependence on caregivers and family for physical care, coupled with a lack of privacy, can be devastating to the adolescent's developing autonomy. Often the adolescent will cope with this forced dependency by displaying maladaptive coping mechanisms such as hostility, aggression, and even treatment refusal.

Besides the worry of their own illness, their self-esteem and identity, adolescents with life-threatening illnesses are concerned about the welfare of their own immediate family. They express concern about the mental health of their parents and siblings, well aware of the burdens and strains under which these other family members must operate.[5]

Changes in mobility and physical appearance, such as those found in adolescents with physical disabilities related to their illnesses, may influence perception of self-worth and social acceptance. It has been demonstrated that physically handicapped seriously ill adolescents score lower on instruments measuring social acceptance and global self-worth.[6]

When the routine of medications, clinic appointments, blood tests, and other required procedures overwhelm an adolescent, he or she may need to distance oneself from the treatment regimen for awhile. A "break" from the constant reminder of the illness is sometimes beneficial. Caregivers need to be aware of this need and to provide such opportunities whenever possible.

Supportive interventions that focus on the promotion of independence and preservation of autonomy will enable the adolescent to accept physical and emotional support without feeling threatened. A sense of being in control can be fostered by offering the adolescent options, whenever they exist.

Adolescents can be a strong source of support for each other. There is a sense of familiarity and acceptance among those sharing a common adversity. Adolescents can be encouraged to expand their network of support through participation in peer groups and other programs developed for this age group. Groups diminish the adolescent's sense of isolation while providing a safe, supportive environment that participants believe in and respond to through mutual disclosure of emotions and experiences. The group normalizes the adolescent's crises and taps into new sources of strength and hope.

COMMUNICATING WITH THE YOUNG CHILD

A recent study reports that less information about diagnosis and treatment of life-threatening illnesses is shared with young children in comparison to children over 9 years of age. This lack of communication may result from the parents' theory that limited disclosure will spare young children from emotional arousal. If this is indeed the goal, it is apparently not achieved in the long term. Over time, young children report experiencing as much disruption and distress from the illness as do their older, more informed counterparts.[7]

The daily lives and routines of children with serious illnesses change in undesirable ways perceptible even to the very young. It is possible that symptoms and treatments of illness may indicate much more powerfully the seriousness of the situation than any words adults may convey or conceal. It is also possible that the lack of disclosure and openness in communication with young children is reflective of the fact that the subject is extremely difficult for parents to address. They may be so emotionally distraught that they are unable to talk with the child about the illness and its implications.

When effective, consistent parent-child communication does take place, it has been demonstrated to positively affect both the coping strategies of the child during treatment[8] and those of the parents after the child's death.[9]

Those communicating with a seriously ill child are often concerned about using the appropriate words. As important as words are, what is most important are the feelings imparted to the child.[10]

For young children, as well as children of all ages, it is important to be observant of nonverbal cues and symbolic language. Children can communicate their feelings through the use of symbolism, as illustrated by a seriously ill 2½-year-old boy. In a play therapy session, while playing jungle with a collection of stuffed animals, he was asked what kind of animal he wanted to be. His reply indicated that he was aware of the gravity of his situation. He answered that he did not want to be any kind of animal at all; he just wanted to grow up and be a big boy.[11]

Young children often respond to encouragement from adults to draw pictures to depict feelings. Expressions of sadness, helplessness, anger, and isolation may be more easily shared in discussions related to drawings that children create than in direct dialogue.[12]

> As Cindy, a terminally ill 3½-year-old girl, grew weaker in her end-stage disease, Sandra, her mother, observed that her daughter demanded her company constantly. Cindy was apprehensive if her mother left her for even a brief period. Cindy would hug her mother many times during the day, hold her tightly, and whisper, "I love you, Mommy."
>
> Sandra asked the nursing staff for material to read to prepare her for her child's death. One evening Sandra was sitting in bed, reading an article given to her by the staff. Cindy lay beside her mother, sleeping. Unable to shield her distress as she read about the needs of dying children, Sandra found herself crying silently. Feeling a hand brush her cheek, she looked down, to find Cindy gazing up at her. "It's alright, Mommy," Cindy said, patting her shoulder. Sandra later told the nursing staff that she felt Cindy knew more than her words could ever express.

THE AWARENESS OF THE SCHOOL-AGE CHILD

The discovery that school-age children have thoughts about death, which appear in their fantasies as well as in their play, is not a new finding. It has been demonstrated that these children experience feelings of grief, fear, loss, and separation.[13] The seriously ill school-age child needs to be able to express fears and concerns in order to decrease anxiety and reduce feelings of isolation and alienation. Current research indicates that children's concepts of death are influenced by their developmental levels, a fact that has implications for those intervening with terminally ill children.

Caregivers may tend to underestimate the dying child's awareness and therefore experience difficulty maintaining a relationship with the child because of their own anxieties.[14] It is imperative that those who work with seriously ill children and their families develop an awareness of their own feelings about life, illness, death, and bereavement. Unless this is accomplished, one cannot be truly therapeutic as a care provider.[15]

Dying children are capable of talking about death.[16] It has been suggested that the best explanations for school-age children are those that are simple, direct, and developmentally appropriate (Table 3.2).

THE DEATH OF A CHILD

The impending death of a child affects the family, as well as community members and the health-care team. Emotional support and education of the family and child are vital for a preparation for the impending death. A

Table 3.2   Guidelines to Be Used When Explaining Death to Children

---

1. Children are ready and capable of talking about anything within their own experience.
2. Use the language of the child.
3. Don't expect an immediate and obvious response from the child.
4. Be a good listener and observer.
5. Be available; don't try to do it all in one discussion.
6. One of the most valuable methods of teaching children about death is to allow them to talk freely and ask their own questions.

Source: Guidelines based on Lonetto R: Children's conceptions of death. New York, Springer, 1980.

common complaint of children and families is that the extensive teaching regarding the diagnosis, preparation for procedures, treatments, therapy, and surgery, and emotional support all decrease significantly as death becomes more imminent. Teaching the family what to expect throughout the terminal and dying process can provide more support and cooperation, as well as make the death of a child an experience in living. The dying process can then be a living experience. The appropriate preparation is not only for the dying process, but is a preparation for the lifetime of grief, healing, and recovery that the family faces.[17]

The dying child should be an active participant in the dying process, depending on his or her age, maturation, and condition. Often family members and staff evade honest communication with the dying child, projecting their own fears and concerns, allegedly making it "easier" for the child. However, children of all ages must attend to unfinished business. Failure to openly communicate with them can thwart their efforts to complete their own tasks.

Kübler-Ross has stated that children are not afraid of death—they are afraid of abandonment. When surrounded with love, joy, and hope, children hold on to their fragile lives.[18]

The grief experienced by a dying child and his or her family is present, even when the family experiences a "good" day. There are ever-present fears and concerns, which need to be explored. Parents often describe their own feelings in relation to how well their child is doing. On a "good" day, a parent may feel encouraged and hopeful. On a "bad" day a parent may be depressed, frightened, and irritable.

The child's emotional state may be labile, with unpredictable mood swings. Families often find it difficult to deal with the child's lability, become impatient, and, subsequently, feel guilty. The child's anger is often expressed with family members, but suppressed with others. Some children are generally irritable with everyone.

The child may behave in many different ways. He or she may be negative, obstinate, and have frequent temper tantrums. Families are often hesitant to impose limits with the seriously ill child, feeling that it is unfair and unkind. In contrast, however, children of all ages feel more secure when appropriate limits are maintained by the adults in their environment, and often respond with a calmer affect.

Some children are overactive, engaging frenetically in social interaction with peers and others with whom they share meaningful relationships. Other children may withdraw from social interaction, spending time alone at home in their rooms. The withdrawal may be appropriate depression or processing of the fact that the individual is indeed dying.

A child's behavior and emotional responses are often the expression of an internal dialogue. There may be evidence that the child is feeling guilty in relation to the diagnosis and illness. The inability to sleep may indicate that he or she is processing fears of death or problems related to the diagnosis. It is essential to know what the child understands about the situation, whether family members and others are allowing the child to discuss what he or she is processing, and whether he or she is indeed discussing this with others.

Toward the end of the terminal phase of the disease, mental faculties and defenses are often weakened. A child may have difficulty concentrating and making decisions. This may be frightening and upsetting to the child and the family. It may not be until this point that the child and family begin to deal with the emotional impact of dying.

THE SPIRITUAL DIMENSION

Even very young children will engage in discussions of what they think dying and the afterlife are like. The family's and the child's beliefs need to be respected, and it is important to be aware of these concepts as held by each member of the family.

In the terminal phase of illness, the dying child completes unfinished business. This may include delegating who will receive what belongings, writing poems or letters, and engaging in dialogue with significant people. Children of all ages have a need to be remembered; they want to be assured that they will not be forgotten by those with whom they have shared their lives.

THE ADOLESCENT AND DEATH

Dying during adolescence is a painfully complex process. While endeavoring to accomplish developmental tasks, the young person must attempt to communicate wishes and needs, decide how to live what life is left, how to prepare family and friends, and how to say good-bye.[19]

The adolescent's orientation toward the future makes the acceptance of personal death especially difficult. Yet dying does not remove the adolescent's desire to strive for independence, but the deteriorating physical condition forces reliance on family and hospital personnel. Dying does not minimize the adolescent's need to control some aspect of his or her life. Trying to make sense of the experience is one way of coping that helps to obtain some level of intellectual control over a painful, difficult reality. Even though dying involves many physical, social, emotional, and symbolic losses, the adolescent keeps struggling to maintain a sense of identity, dignity, and pride.

In order to cope with the anxiety elicited by thoughts of their own mortality, some adolescents use denial. Some will discuss their dying openly with family, friends, and health-care professionals, while others will not. Some adolescents protect their families by sharing with others. Many who are aware that they are dying want confirmation from a caregiver.

All seriously ill adolescents are preoccupied at some point during their illness with the crucial question "Why me?" This query is an adaptive reaction through which they develop a personal theory to justify their experience. Adolescents tend to believe that everything happens because of a special reason. Once they have discovered the reason, they feel more in control of their own lives.

The will to live can coexist with an awareness of the possibility of death.[20] All seriously ill adolescents know at some level that they are dying, but they fluctuate between awareness and denial. Knowing that death is a reality does not mean that they accept death. Adolescents often experience a great deal of anxiety that is related more to the process of dying than to death itself.

Often adolescents use symbolic language to communicate their feelings and concerns related to death.[20] These may be related in stories or drawings and need to be understood in order to relate meaningfully with the individual.

Coexisting with the need to maintain a sense of belonging is the adolescent's need to withdraw emotionally as death approaches. The need to belong and maintain a place among friends and family does not waiver, even during the dying process.

Some adolescents assume a supportive and protective role toward significant people in their lives, or strive to achieve major accomplishments in an effort to maintain a sense of belonging in the face of impending death. Others, afraid of being abandoned by loved ones, secure the attention of those around them by assuming the role of victim of their circumstances.

Adolescents withdraw emotionally as death approaches. This distancing provides the opportunity to conserve energy to focus on a few significant relationships, rather than dealing with multiple painful separations.[21]

> Jane, at 17, was an assertive adolescent who had been diagnosed with osteosarcoma at age 14. Her battle with disease resulted in a right above-the-knee amputation, yet the illness continued to progress despite aggressive treatment.
>
> One of the most distressing aspects of serious illness for Jane was the fact that her family was unable to hear her decision to discontinue chemotherapy. Both her parents and her younger sister insisted that she not "give up," and continued to search for alternative treatment options. Jane firmly expressed a desire to leave the hospital and return home to be with her best friends.
>
> A care conference composed of members of the multidisciplinary team was held at Jane's bedside when she found herself lacking the strength to move to the conference room. Once more she stated her wishes, and once again her family desperately pleaded with her to reconsider. The team encouraged the family to listen carefully to what Jane was asking.
>
> Jane's family finally consented to take her home, where she was reunited with three close friends who had been her companions since early childhood. She died in her bed, at home, three days later.

Active listening on the part of caregivers provides adolescents with a forum to express feelings of anger and loss. Optimism can be maintained throughout the dying process if the adolescent can be assisted to focus on the present moment, give meaning to his or her experiences, and preserve a sense of dignity and self-respect.

In terminal illness, the family, not the patient alone, is considered the unit of care. Support for the family is critical when the dying patient is a child. It has been determined that the loss of a child produces higher grief intensities in the survivors than either the loss of a spouse or a parent.[22] Kübler-Ross emphasizes that caregivers cannot truly help the terminally ill child or adolescent unless they include the family.[21] It is therefore essential that the dying process be discussed in terms of how it will affect each person involved.

NOTES

1. Petrillo M, Sanger S: Emotional care of hospitalized children. Philadelphia, Lippincott, 1980.

2. Biehler, RF: Psychology applied to teaching. Boston, Houghton Mifflin, 1974.

3. Ellis, J: Coping with adolescent cancer: It's a matter of adaptation. J Assoc Pediatr Oncol Nurs 8:10–17, 1991.

4. Blotcky, AD, Cohen DG: Psychological assessment of the adolescent with cancer. J Assoc Pediatr Oncol Nurs 2:8–14, 1985.

5. Chesler, M: Surviving childhood cancer: The struggle goes on. J Assoc Pediatr Oncol Nurs 7:57–59, 1990.

6. Hockenberry-Eaton, M, Cotanch, P: Evaluation of a child's perceived self-competence during treatment for cancer. J Pediatr Oncol Nurs 6:55–62, 1989.

7. Claflin, C, Barbarin, O: Does "telling" less protect more? Relationships among age, information disclosure, and what children with cancer see and feel. J Ped Psychol 16:169–191, 1991.

8. Spinetta JJ, Maloney LS: The child with cancer: Patterns of communication and denial. J Consult Clin Psychol 46:1540–1541, 1978.

9. Spinetta JJ, Swarmer JA, Sheposh JP: Effective parental coping following the death of a child from cancer. J Pediatr Psychol 6:261–263, 1981.

10. Foley GV, Whittam EH: Care of the child dying of cancer: Part 1. Ca—A Cancer J for Clinicians 40:327–351, 1990.

11. Adams-Greenly, M: Helping children communicate about serious illness and death. J Psychosocial Oncol 2:61–72, 1984.

12. Gibbons, MB: A child dies, a child survives: The impact of sibling loss. J Pediatr Health Care 6:65–72, 1992.

13. Anthony S: The child's discovery of death: A study of child psychology. New York, Harcourt, Brace, and World, 1940.

14. Gibbons MB: When the dying patient is a child: A challenge for the living. In MJ Hockenberry and DC Coody (Eds), Pediatric oncology and hematology perspectives on care. St. Louis, C. V. Mosby, 1986.

15. Gibbons, MB: Coping with childhood cancer: A family perspective. In PW Power, AE Dell Orto, and MB Gibbons (Eds), Family interventions throughout chronic illness and disability. New York, Springer, 1988.

16. Koocher G: Talking with children about death. Am J Orthopsychiatry 44:404–411, 1974.

17. Gyulay, J: Home care for the dying child. Issues in Comprehensive Nurs 12:33–69, 1989.

18. Kübler-Ross, E: On death and dying. New York, Macmillan, 1969.

19. Pazola, K, Gerberg, A: Privileged communication: Talking with a dying adolescent. J Maternal Child Nursing 15:16–21, 1990.

20. Papatadatou, D: Caring for dying adolescents. Nurs Times 85:28–31, 1989.

21. Kübler-Ross, E: On children and death. New York, Macmillan, 1983.

22. Saunders, CC: A comparison of adult bereavement on the death of a spouse, child, and parent. Omega 10:303–320, 1979.

4

Neonatal Death

CHERYL MARCO NAULTY

There are really no "expected deaths" in the newborn nursery. When parents embark on the path of creating a child, they envision a perfect outcome. Anything less is devastating.

Through major advancements in technology and improved understanding of the pathophysiology of certain diseases, many infants, for whom there was no hope of therapy or cure, are now being saved. The majority of neonatal deaths are related to complications of prematurity and congenital anomalies. The reduction in neonatal mortality over the past two decades has been largely because of improved survival for low birthweight infants. Before 1970, fewer than 10% extremely low birthweight infants (<1000g, <28 weeks gestational age [GA]) survived compared with more than 50% in the 1980s.[1] Even infants with major congenital abnormalities or significant perinatal events, for whom death was the only option, may now be offered lifesaving interventions.

Along with the increase in neonatal survival, there is also an increased concern about the long-term morbidity of some of the survivors (Figure 4.1). The rate of serious long-term disability increases with decreasing birthweight. Many infants continue to suffer from lifelong, handicapping conditions such as chronic cardiopulmonary disease, short bowel syndrome, or various manifestations of brain damage. One-fourth of very low birthweight survivors (<1500g, <32 weeks GA) will have major neurodevelopmental impairments, and far more present at school age with specific learning disabilities and lower cognitive scores than their full-term counterparts.[2]

As advanced technology and refinements in care continue to improve survival for these infants, questions regarding the lower limits of viability must be considered. It is becoming increasingly apparent that certain biological limitations cannot and may not ever be overcome. There is a danger that the issue of the patient as the focus of treatment may be swallowed up by the new technology.[3] Certainly if new and more aggressive therapies

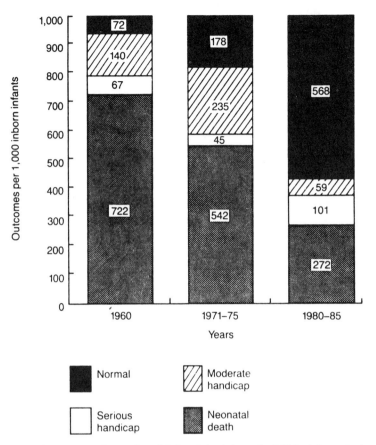

Figure 4.1 Outcomes of very low birthweight infants (< 1500 g) born in level III hospitals from 1960 to 1985. (From Health Technology Case Study 38: Neonatal Intensive Care for Low Birthweight Infants: Costs and Effectiveness. Washington, D.C., Congress of United States Office of Technology Assessment, 1987; with permission.)

had not been applied to the smaller and sicker infants of the past two decades, much of the improvement in neonatal mortality would not have taken place. However, once this "machinery" has been set in place, it often becomes difficult to stop. To preserve life at all costs and to use "the uncontrolled application of medical technology may be detrimental to individuals and families."[3] While consideration ought to be given to the initiation of aggressive treatment, there may also be a place for the withdrawal or the withholding of extraordinary measures. In addition, it needs to be made clear to both the family and health-care professionals that, from an ethical, decision-making standpoint, there is no distinction between withdrawing treatment and withholding treatment altogether.

MAKING DECISIONS IN THE INTENSIVE CARE NURSERY

At first glance, the application of hospice principles in the neonatal inten-sive care setting appears to be an oxymoron; that is, consideration of hos-pice and the acceptance of death seem like foreign concepts in the high-tech, life-sustaining atmosphere of an intensive care nursery. Much of this im-pression is based on the multiplicity of factors that must be considered when making the decision on how long treatment can or should be continued. In addition to the medical facts, legal and ethical concerns, financial issues, socioemotional experiences, and cultural bias all influence the attitudes and opinions of the family and staff when approaching this kind of decision.

Medical Considerations in Decision Making

In the field of medicine, precedent for determining criteria for withholding treatment is based on the assumption that physicians have precise knowl-edge concerning outcome, which is often not the case. In the neonatal intensive care unit (NICU), the inability to reliably predict long-term prog-nosis in all circumstances and the uncertainty of the quality of life, if long-term disability seems a certainty, cloud the issues when making decisions. It is often not clear where to draw the line between ordinary and extraordi-nary care. Much of the therapy in a neonatal intensive care unit might be considered "experimental," as the technology proven beneficial for more mature infants is applied to the smaller and less mature.

What the Laws Say: The Baby Doe Regulations

There exists a real uncertainty about the legal status of infants, and a distinct ambiguity between legal doctrine and clinical practice. The courts have acknowledged the rights of parents to make decisions on behalf of their children but do not consider the right absolute.[4] Nor have the courts been persuaded that quality of life considerations should be decisive.[4] Car-rying the interpretation of the law to the letter, Robertson[5] has written that parents, who withhold ordinary lifesaving medical treatment from a newborn, are liable for prosecution under state homicide or child abuse statutes. This liability extends as well to physicians and other care providers and hospital officials.

In 1984 the federal government enacted legislation that was designed to curtail the practice of "infanticide" by the medical profession. Four signifi-cant events over the years prior to 1984 had enabled this legislation to come about.[6] Early in 1973, Congress authorized funding to study child abuse and to help states set up agencies to deal with this problem. Later that same year, Congress passed the Rehabilitation Act of 1973 that contained a section prohibiting providers of medical care from discrimination against the handicapped. Both laws provided the framework for future amendments aimed at the withholding or the withdrawal of care from sick newborns. The third event was rooted in the Supreme Court's *Roe vs. Wade* decision regarding abortion. Arguments, similar to the antiabortion perspective pertaining to the sanctity of life, resurfaced regarding the termination of life based on a prognosis for poor quality of life. Finally, the publication in the *New England Journal of Medicine* by Duff and Campbell[3] on the use of death as a management option in the NICU set the stage for the public furor surrounding the "Baby Doe" legislation that was to come.

The cases of Baby Doe (1982) and Baby Jane Doe (1983)[4], which gave rise to the public controversy in 1984, both concerned the rights of parents to withhold treatment from their handicapped infants. While the specific judgments in each of these cases were procedural and not substantive, the issues that emerged for debate included every person's right to nonheroic, lifesaving, medical intervention; strictures against child abuse based on neglect; parental rights to choose from among all medically valid courses of action for their child; and the need to protect the interests of the child.[4] Following these two specific cases, there was a directive issued from the White House to the Department of Health and Human Services for guidelines consistent with current law for nontreatment decisions.[4,6] This resulted in two efforts on the part of the federal government to establish these guidelines.

A directive was sent out to federally supported hospitals under Section 504 of the Rehabilitation Act of 1973. This law states that hospitals would be in violation of the federal law if they withheld any ordinary benefit or service from handicapped citizens, simply based on the handicapping condition. The directive broadened the scope of the law to include treatment or nourishment of handicapped infants, saying that it is unlawful for a recipient of federal financial assistance to withhold from a handicapped infant nutritional sustenance or medical or surgical treatment required to correct a life-threatening condition, if (1) the withholding is based on the fact that the infant is handicapped; and (2) the handicap does not render the treatment or nutritional sustenance contraindicated.[4] To ensure compliance, it called for the establishment of twenty-four-hour hotlines to receive complaints and the famous "Baby Doe Squads" to investigate alleged violations. This directive was overturned in the U.S. District Court of Appeals based on the original intent of Section 504, which was to assure the disabled equality in areas such as housing and employment and not to compel the treatment of handicapped infants.[7] The important long-term outcome of this legislative battle was the acknowledgment by the Department of Health and Human Services of the rights of physicians to make reasonable medical judgments for their patients.[4]

The second pertinent piece of legislation to emerge out of this period was the 1984 amendment to the Child Abuse Prevention and Treatment Act, which is still currently in place. Under this legislation, the traditional scope of child abuse is broadened to include medical neglect. Medical neglect is herein defined as including the withholding of medically indicated treatment from a disabled infant with a life-threatening condition.[4,6] The withholding of medically indicated treatment is further defined as "the failure to respond to the infant's life-threatening condition by providing treatment which, in the treating physician's reasonable medical judgement, will be most likely to be effective in ameliorating or correcting all such conditions." There are three exceptions: (1) the infant is chronically and irreversibly comatose; (2) the provision of such treatment would merely prolong dying, not be effective in ameliorating or correcting all of the infant's life-threatening conditions, or otherwise be futile in terms of survival of the infant; and (3) the provision of such treatment would be virtually futile in terms of the survival of the infant, and the treatment itself under such circumstances would be inhumane.[4] By enacting this law, the federal government has taken the position that viability alone mandates treatment no matter what the quality of life might be.

The law also introduced guidelines for the establishment of Infant Care Review Committees or Bioethics Committees at all health-care institutions. The purpose of these committees is not to make binding decisions but to set policy, review individual cases, and offer advice to the treating physician on request. The end result of all of this legislation is that, within certain guidelines, physicians and parents together are empowered with the ability to make choices for the infant. Guidance may be sought from a Bioethics Committee, but the advice is not binding. Finally, this approach exerts a great deal of pressure on judgments about prognosis.

Concerns of the Family

To turn now to issues relating directly to families, multiple factors may influence parents' attitudes toward making a decision for hospice and the acceptance of their current loss.[8] What prior losses have they experienced, either through abortion, stillbirth, or another neonatal death, or the loss of another family member through death or divorce? What is their degree of prenatal attachment to this pregnancy? Was it a wanted or planned pregnancy? What were their preconceived expectations of the pregnancy and birth and of this infant's future?

The suddenness of the current loss might not allow sufficient time to adjust to the severity of the problem and the differences between their expectations and reality. Cultural differences influence the response to death and dying and overt expressions of grief. Personal strengths strongly affect the reactions and decision-making abilities of the family. Whether there are strong support structures through extended family, friends, or formal religious groups, a stable relationship between parents, financial stability, or freedom from other outside pressures, all impact on the family's ability to cope with the current crisis.

Financial Issues

Although financial concerns do not and should not play a role in the decision to withhold or withdraw treatment in the nursery, questions are being raised about the ultimate cost and the cost-effectiveness of neonatal intensive care. In an era where the price of health care is rising annually and represents approximately 12% of the Gross National Product in the United States, the dollars spent on neonatal intensive care loom large. Neonatal intensive care is expensive and the numbers increase as birthweight falls. The incremental cost of care to produce a survivor in 1984 was $86,000 for infants with birthweights between 1000 and 1500 grams and $118,000 for infants with birthweights below 1000 grams.[1] The charges for the sickest and tiniest infants rank with the most expensive medical procedures performed today. "The worth of a life saved, however, is ultimately a value judgement involving ethical and social considerations. The results from cost-effectiveness studies alone cannot guide decisions regarding who should receive care."[1]

THE GRIEF PROCESS IN THE NEONATAL INTENSIVE CARE UNIT

No matter how enormous the monetary outlay is for neonatal intensive care, the dollars represent only a small portion of the total "cost" in emotional grief and pain experienced by the families as well as the nursery staff. Parents expect a normal, healthy, full-term infant and are not prepared for dealing with an outcome that is anything less than that. The variance between preconceived "fantasy" and reality determines the magnitude of feelings of loss.[9] Parents must first mourn the loss of the perfect child and then reattach to the real child.

Parental Grief

For the grieving process and the decision for hospice to work, the parents must be in synchrony with one another. Yet the perceptions and responses of fathers versus mothers may be quite different. Aside from cultural variations in male and female expressions of grief, there are unique circumstances in the NICU that may magnify these differences.[8] While mothers often have bonded to the child during the pregnancy, fathers may experience a psychological lag in investment because of their lack of physiological involvement during the pregnancy. Fathers, in turn, may become increasingly more attached after delivery as they witness the resuscitation and accompany the baby to the nursery or on the transport. The father may become the foremost champion of the infant and the primary source of information for the hospitalized mother, who may be physically separated from her infant for days. This role may force the father to be stoic and protective of the mother, further suppressing his own emotional responses. The fact that the intensive care setting is often in a tertiary hospital distant from the family's home, with care delivered by new and unfamiliar physicians, magnifies the problem.

Parents, who are experiencing neonatal loss, have special needs and unique reactions that must be understood by the neonatal staff.[10] As there is no "formula" for grieving, misdirected anger has to be understood and support must be nonjudgmental. Parents may require complete and detailed information about their infant and the reasoning behind the care given. Rather than being regarded as a challenge to the caregivers, parental need for information may be their way of coping, particularly with the uncertainty of the outcome. Parents' processing and understanding of information can be one way for them to regain some control and to participate in events that will have a lifelong impact. Continuity and consistency in communication is vital, as each parent may hear and process the same information differently. The physicians and neonatal staff need to provide a realistic picture of the infant's illness and prognosis. The family may understand at some level how serious the situation is but need someone among the professionals to openly acknowledge the severity. An overly optimistic approach may be more cruel in the long term and may delay the grieving process, and ultimately, the acceptance of death. The role of the professional staff in the decision-making process needs to remain interpersonal, intimate, humane, respectful, and sensitive to long-term emotional concerns.[11]

Although the grief process in the NICU is most often associated with the death of an infant, the survival of a handicapped child can bring chronic sorrow to a family. Even though they may accept and adjust to the defects, they will continue to mourn for the loss of the perfect child. Chronic sorrow can be a reaction to the daily stresses of coping with the handicapping condition and is a constant reminder of what the child is not.[8]

Grieving and the Professional Staff

Professionals also need to deal with their own feelings of grief and loss, especially after repeatedly experiencing it. Since neonatal intensive care has been so successful, physicians, particularly, may feel a sense of failure and powerlessness when talking about death.[11] The personal feelings, attitudes, and biases of the professional staff may affect their ability to deal with and be supportive of the family. Avoidance of the family or of directly addressing their own feelings may make the family's ability to cope with the death and grieving more difficult.[8] It is important for the staff to establish their own support structure, either formal or informal, as a mechanism to work through their own feelings.

HOSPICE IN THE NEONATAL INTENSIVE CARE UNIT

In order for a hospice program to be successful in a neonatal intensive care setting, major changes in the traditional orientation of the medical staff are necessary and alternatives to the noisy, high tech environment must be available. A room filled with machines, fluid-filled tubes, and beeping monitors is hardly conducive to quiet intimacy with a dying infant. The mind set of the staff is to view survival as the only acceptable goal and death as a failure. They are the ones in charge of the infant and in control of the outcome, even though the parents may participate in some routine care tasks and are consulted regarding therapeutic options.

For hospice to work in the NICU, both hospital personnel and family must adapt the hospice principles to this setting by initiating less active forms of therapy, creating a more comfortable environment, and shifting the focus from the patient to the family.[12] Active cooperation and participation of the nursing staff are essential for creating the right environment for hospice. The nurses must be educated in the concept that, while death may be a tragedy, it does not necessarily imply a failure. Thinking becomes refocused from curative to palliative. With this mind set the staff can then help the family make the decision for dying, "allowing the decision to be a process, allowing anticipatory grief."[13] Both the staff and parents can then become proxies for the dying infant, who cannot speak for him or herself. This attitude generates a strong and caring bond with the family and a supportive, permissive environment conducive to expressing feelings.

Often the family cannot perform all the care as in adult hospice. The nursery staff should allow as much family participation in the infant's care as possible.[14] Touching and holding the infant is especially important, if it can be done without any tubes, wires, or monitors attached. The nursing staff must achieve a balance between the willingness to provide care and support and to share the experience with the family, while allowing the family private time and space as often as needed. Taking a picture of the infant during this time may provide lasting memories.[8,12]

The physical environment of an NICU is unfriendly and intimidating. Hospice requires a comfortable, more homelike environment separate from the NICU. The setting should be a separate room with comfortable chairs, which allows for privacy, yet still needs to be adjacent to the NICU, so the family will not feel isolated.[14,15]

The last, essential component for a successful hospice program is a mechanism for follow-up after death.[12,15] Some programs will contact the parents after several months just to learn how well they are coping or to discuss the autopsy. Learning the results of the autopsy can be very important. Knowing how or why the baby died may resolve lingering issues of grief or guilt. This follow-up often brings the family back into contact with the professionals some months after the death, at a time when grieving may still be real and fresh but support structures still not in place. This contact may afford an opportunity for assessment, counseling, and referral, if needed.

Although few neonatal intensive care units have reported formal hospice programs,[14] the application of this approach to the dying infant is more widespread. The attending physician will work to establish collaborative parent-physician discussions with active involvement of the related medical team. Even without dedicated space, efforts are readily made to afford the family the privacy and intimacy required. Most important is the recognition that this is "a process built on trust and requiring time, information, honesty, and empathy."[11]

The issue of death in the nursery is a complex one, one not easily answered by rules or regulations, legal or ethical arguments, medical facts, or emotional pleas. While the medical profession must continue to search for new cures and seek ways to apply technological advances to the care of these infants, it cannot lose sight of its primary responsibility—the welfare of the child. "We are on more humane ground when we base our treatment decisions on what is in the child's best interest. This, of course, is not the end of the matter, because what is best for the child is often far from clear. But we are at least on the right track when we make compassion for the child our sole standard."[7]

NOTES

1. U.S. Congress, Office of Technology Assessment: Neonatal intensive care for low birthweight infants: costs and effectiveness. Health Technol Case Study 38, p 4, Washington, D.C., U. S. Congress, 1987.

2. The Infant Health and Development Program. Enhancing the outcomes of low-birth-weight, premature infants; a multisite, randomized trial. JAMA 263: 3035–3042, 1990.

3. Duff RS, Campbell AGM: Moral and ethical dilemmas in the special care nursery. N Engl J Med 289:890–894, 1973.

4. Moreno JD: Ethical and legal issues in the care of the impaired newborn. Clin Perinatol 14:345–360, 1987.

5. Robertson JA, Fost N: Passive euthanasia of defective newborn infants: legal considerations. J Pediatr 88:883–889, 1976.

6. Lund N: Infanticide, physicians, and the law: the "Baby Doe" amendments to the child abuse prevention and treatment act. Am J Law Med 11:1–29, 1985.

7. Lyon J: Playing God in the nursery. New York, W W Norton, 1985.

8. Gardner SL, Merenstein GB: Helping families deal with perinatal loss. Neonatal Network/October:17–33, 1986.

9. Gardner SL, Merenstein GB: Perinatal grief and loss; an overview. Neonatal Network/October:7–15, 1986.

10. Eikner S: Dealing with long-term problems: a parent's perspective. Neonatal Network/October:45–49, 1986.

11. Jellinek MS, Catlin EA, Todres ID, Cassem EH: Facing tragic decisions with parents in the neonatal intensive care unit: clinical perspectives. Pediatr 89:119–122, 1992.

12. Harmon FJ, Glicken AD, Siegel RE: Neonatal loss in the ICN: effects of maternal grieving and a program for intervention. J Am Aca Child Psychiatry 23: 68–71, 1984.

13. Butler NC: The NICU culture vs the hospice culture; can they mix? Neonatal Network/October:35–42, 1986.

14. Whitfield JM, Siegel RE, Glicken AD, Harmon RJ, Powers LK, Goldson EJ: The application of hospice concepts to neonatal care. Am J Dis Child 136:421–424, 1982.

15. Landon-Malone KA, Kirkpatrick JM, Stull SP: Incorporating hospice care in a community hospital NICU. Neonatal Network/October:113–119, 1986.

5

Care for the Child with HIV Infection and AIDS

LORI WIENER, CINDY FAIR, and PHILIP A. PIZZO

During the past decade, the incidence of HIV infection in children has been increasing rapidly. Indeed AIDS has already become among the top disease-specific causes of death in children and in some parts of the United States. For example, in certain areas of New Jersey, AIDS has become the leading cause of death in children who are less than 4 years of age. In the United States, between 1500–2000 children who have been infected with HIV are being born each year. As the numbers of women of childbearing age increases each year, it is likely that this annual incidence will also increase. In comparison, it is notable that in the United States approximately 6500–7200 children are diagnosed with cancer each year. However, thanks to medical research, more than half of these children are potentially curable of their cancer. Unfortunately, no cure exists for HIV infection and at this time it must be anticipated that every infected child will eventually die as a consequence of this infection. On a worldwide basis, the figures are even more startling, since it is estimated that there will be more than 10 million HIV-infected children by the end of this decade. Overall, the greatest impact will be in racial minority groups in the United States and in children in developing nations. Virtually all of the current and future cases of HIV infection in infants and children result from vertical transmission from an infected mother.

The course of HIV infection is often dramatically accelerated in children compared to adults with the majority of those with vertically acquired HIV infection becoming symptomatic within the first 2 years of life. Also, the clinical presentation of HIV infection can differ from that in adults. For example, recurrent bacterial infections can be a serious problem for children, along with many of the opportunistic infections (e.g., *Pneumocystis carinii* pneumonia) observed in adults. One of the most devastating aspects of HIV infection in children is its impact on the central nervous system. Indeed, from 50 to 90% of children appear to develop neurodevelopmental abnormalities, most frequently manifested as motor deficits, the delayed acquisition or loss of normal developmental milestones (e.g., walking, speech, self-care skills), and cognitive deficits. Symptoms can develop and progress rapidly or continue to evolve over time. In addition to affecting the central nervous system, HIV infection can also impact adversely on the growth of children as well as in damage to vital organs, including the heart, lungs, kidneys, and liver. Clearly HIV infection represents a multisystem disorder in children, with the potential for repetitive life-threatening events. The clinical course can progress rapidly or over years of time. Even with medical intervention, however, HIV infection is inevitably fatal in children at this time. Surely the last several years has witnessed considerable progress, both in the supportive care of children and treatment of intercurrent infectious and noninfectious complications, but also in the introduction of agents designed to impact on the HIV virus itself. These antiretroviral drugs, such as azidothymidine (AZT), dideoxycytidine (ddC), dideoxyinosine (ddI) have contributed to improvements in the quality and duration of life of children with HIV infection. The emphasis at this time must be on the development of strategies or regimens that will further improve the survival of children with HIV infection. But hope must be tempered by reality, and attention to the dignity of both the life and death of children with HIV infection must be the concern of health-care providers. Hospice is a renowned concept in providing just this type of dignified care to the dying.

Historical Response of Hospice to Pediatric AIDS

Historically, hospice has been a primary support to terminally ill children and their families. In general, hospices are accepting children with HIV into their care. However, some hospices have criteria for accepting children into their programs that are problematic for infected children and their families. For example, children who are receiving AZT or Total Parenteral Nutrition (TPN) may not be accepted because these treatments may be considered life prolonging or curative. In children with HIV infection, however, these therapies should be viewed as palliative rather than curative. Some hospice programs will only provide service to those children who have been given a defined amount of time to live. This can present problems to a family dealing with HIV since it can be difficult to clearly predict the life expectancy of a child with HIV. Not all children with AIDS are afforded the opportunity to die at home. Because of the unpredictable nature of HIV disease, children are often suddenly stricken with an acute illness that becomes fatal while the child is still hospitalized rather than at home.

The AIDS epidemic has posed a special challenge to hospice caregivers (Table 5.1). Nationwide, there is an increasing number of families in need of hospice services. When an entire family is infected, hospice workers may be serving more than one family member at a time. Both of these factors call for new and creative approaches to service delivery and the need to examine existing policies that may appear inflexible. The demand for hospice services will only increase as the number of infected family members rises. Hospice can play a vital role in providing comprehensive care to children and families with AIDS.

The management of the child with HIV infection must also be approached within the context of the families and communities. Accordingly, we will address some of the factors that must be considered in developing an optimal care plan for the child with HIV infection, focusing particularly on unique social issues.

SOCIAL CONSIDERATIONS AFFECTING THE CARE OF THE HIV-INFECTED CHILD

Family Constellation

Pediatric AIDS most often is a family disease and the child is frequently the index case to the indentification of other infected family members. Pediatric HIV infection often affects families who are already socially and emotion-

Table 5.1   Unique Social Challenges in the Care of Children with AIDS

- Family disease
- Exposure to drug use, drug culture
- Minority representation
- Adolescents at risk
- Stigmatization
- Discrimination
- Fears associated with disclosure
- Secrecy, isolation
- Difficulty accessing existing support services
- Bureaucratic challenges

ally disenfranchised.[1] The primary caretaker is commonly a single parent who must rely on public welfare programs that are inadequate for a family whose child suffers from a chronic and debilitating illness.[2]

As a parent becomes too ill or becomes unable to care for his or her HIV-infected child, relatives and extended family may be called on for support. In these instances caretaking responsibilities may be shared among family members. A common pattern that is emerging in families is that more and more grandparents are being called on to care for their sick children as well as their infected grandchildren. Unfortunately, it is not always possible for a child to remain with its family of origin. In cases where families are unwilling or unable to provide support, foster care becomes the only alternative.

The Need For Permanence

HIV-infected children may move to and from foster homes or from one chaotic system to another due to parental incarceration, addiction, illness, abandonment, court removal, hospitalization, or homelessness.[3] The lack of appropriate foster homes, in-home programs, and hospice care in certain communities has resulted in some HIV-infected children remaining hospitalized for as long as two years in acute care hospitals when their conditions no longer required hospitalization.[4] Early planning is essential to prevent further chaos and to develop stable home environments for these children who face physical and familial devastation.

There are, however, several potential obstacles to the provision of a permanent home for these children, including the emphasis the child welfare field has traditionally made for family cohesion (reunification). Ideally, children should spend their lives with their biological family. However, illness, drug use, neglect, or abuse may make this impossible or not in the child's best interest. During the months to years of waiting to see whether reunification can take place, the child is left with an uncertain future. The length and quality of life of HIV-infected children are already uncertain. Separations are stressful and most children already worry about separation from those they love through death. Serious consideration needs to be made toward expediting the placement process. Permanent foster homes can be an extremely rewarding experience for both the child and family. As Brother Toby, an adoptive parent, said:

> There has to be a humane approach to get children freed for permanency—so children can grow up in a permanent, stable home where bonding can take place, where the child owns one of us—so when the time comes for dying they do not reach out to a strange hand. I guess that is the ultimate right of any child—not to die among strangers.[5]

Drug-Dependent Parents

Parental drug use and HIV infection in children are, unfortunately, often linked. Intravenous drug use is the primary route of maternal infection (42% of cases reported from July 1988 to June 1989).[6] However, the number of women who acquired their infection from heterosexual contact with a partner who used intravenous drugs is increasing.[6]

Drug-dependent parents pose a challenge to professionals working with the family of an HIV-infected child. The nature of the difficulties posed include inconsistent compliance to medical treatments, erratic behavior, impaired judgment, resistance to intrusion from "outsiders" in order to protect illicit activities, and extreme emotional lability. Often, protective services must be involved when a child's safety is at stake. In addition, care for such a child requires coordination with multiple agencies.

Drug-using parents of an HIV-infected child may use drugs as a means to anesthetize themselves against the pain and guilt brought about by watching their child, potentially their partner and themselves slowly succumb to illness. A parent who has remained drug free for a period of time may relapse when new developments occur in their own health status or in the health of their child. The chronic nature of addiction should be recognized by caretakers involved with the family. If relapses can be anticipated and appropriate supports provided, crises may be avoided.

Treatment for substance-abusing parents is often difficult to find. There are frequently long waiting lists and few rehabilitation facilities that accept either Medicaid or pregnant women. Most rehabilitation programs do not provide child care for dependent children. It is important to remember that AIDS is currently a disease that primarily affects unempowered minorities: women, children, blacks, Hispanics, homosexuals, and intravenous-drug abusers,[7] many of whom are already burdened with discrimination, poverty, and institutional barriers to treatment when confronted with HIV.

Black and Hispanic Children

Blacks and Hispanics are disproportionately represented among both adult and pediatric AIDS cases. Over 80% of children infected with HIV are from these minority groups. The majority of these children live in deteriorating urban centers. Many families are involved in drug use which, coupled with poverty, minority status, and few social supports, leads to a very compromised environment for children. Access to primary health care is a major problem for families living with HIV. Often families rely on public hospitals which may have limited resources. Families may also have a mistrust of government agencies that stems from generations of difficulties encountered when accessing services.

It is important for care providers involved with minority families to understand cultural beliefs that may impact on health behaviors. In the black community AIDS is a particularly stigmatizing disease. As a result, traditional social supports may not be available during times of stress and illness to black families who are coping with HIV disease.[8] Historically, black churches have rallied to organize communities around illness among its members. However, this has not necessarily occurred for HIV-infected blacks. As a consequence, caregivers will be confronted with socially isolated families who do not have supports normally accessed in times of difficulty.

There are also many cultural values within the Hispanic family to be considered. Language abilities and educational background have an impact on health behavior.[8] Many Hispanics have limited mastery of the English language and have difficulty reading even in their primary language.

In working with the families of HIV-infected Hispanic children, it is important to assess who the significant members of the nuclear and extended family are.[8] It is not uncommon for several generations of a family to be living together in a single dwelling. Family members will often turn to another family member when confronted with a problem rather than ask for outside help. Within a Hispanic family the husband or male in the family has authority over female family members. It is therefore important to consider his opinion when the family is confronted with decisions. There is also an emphasis on fertility and childbearing among Hispanic families. As a result, issues regarding family planning must be approached with cultural sensitivity.

Adolescents

Currently, the prevalence of AIDS among adolescents accounts for less than 1% of all cases of AIDS.[9] However, many young adults with AIDS acquired their infection with HIV during their teenage years. Many HIV-infected teens are from disadvantaged impoverished backgrounds. Adolescents who are alienated from their families of origin have many needs. Runaways are often sex workers, exchanging sexual favors for money or drugs in order to survive on the streets. These youths are at particular risk of HIV infection. Disenfranchised youth may need assistance finding clothing, food, shelter, medical care, and educational or employment opportunities. HIV-infected teens need access to education regarding safer sex practices, drug rehabilitation, and family planning information.

Given the unique psychosocial nature of adolescents, those who are HIV positive present caregivers with new challenges. The special developmental tasks of adolescence are complicated by the course of illness and stigma associated with AIDS. The adolescent is struggling with developing a sense of self that is independent from their family of origin. A diagnosis of HIV infection during the critical time of adolescence can undermine this process. The adolescent is suddenly thrust into a medical setting that may not allow autonomy or may be forced to return to the family and assume a less independent role. In addition, the usual support of a teen's peer relations may not be accessed for fear of rejection or discrimination. Social isolation can be compounded by the actual separation from neighborhood and school necessitated by medical treatment. Patient support and establishing a strong relationship with the adolescent is of the utmost importance when working with teens who are experiencing the effects of stigma.

The Effects of Stigma

The stigma of AIDS affects children and families from diagnosis through the course of illness and beyond. All individuals with HIV infection are at risk for social ostracism. Parents often feel the need to lie to friends and relatives and withhold information from their children for fear of persecution. While a young child may not be cognizant of it, their opportunities may be limited due to institutional and social discrimination. The school-age child and adolescent may feel the direct effects of others' fears and ignorance concerning the disease. As a result, families live in a state of isolation, afraid to share with others what their day-to-day life is like.

The stigma associated with AIDS sets this disease apart from all other contemporary health problems. Even after a child has died some families still feel they have no choice but to continue to lie about their child's illness. The mother of an 8-year-old girl who died over a year ago of AIDS recently began attending support groups for bereaved parents. She is still unable to disclose the diagnosis and told the group members her daughter died of "birth complications." Some families have chosen to be open regarding the HIV diagnosis. Many have received compassion and support. Others have found themselves faced with ostracism and discrimination.

Discrimination

Cases where individuals with HIV infection have been denied basic rights and services on the basis of their illness is most unfortunate. There are medical professionals who have refused to work with HIV-infected individuals. Discrimination is a by-product of fears concerning transmission of the virus and the lethal nature of the infection. Discrimination can occur on many different levels and can range from blatant to subtle. Institutions as well as individuals discriminate against families with HIV infection. Infected children have been expelled from day care, schools, and religious institutions.[10] Families have been evicted from housing and parents have lost jobs when the diagnosis of HIV was uncovered.

There is a rapidly growing body of case law based on court rulings regarding what does and does not constitute discrimination. However, many cases of discrimination are subtle and never reach the national level as the situation of Bobby illustrates. Bobby is an 11-year-old boy with hemophilia and HIV infection. At the beginning of the school year the principal informed Bobby's mother that a nurse, dressed in a white uniform was hired to follow Bobby throughout the school day to prevent other children from coming in contact with Bobby's bodily fluids. After protesting to the school board, Bobby's mother was able to have the nurse removed. Unfortunately subtle discriminatory practices continued. Bobby was required to use only one particular bathroom in the school. No other child was allowed to use the bathroom following Bobby until the bathroom had been cleaned with bleach. HIV-infected children desire and deserve as normal a life as possible. Unfortunately, discriminatory practices as described above only serve to single out the child, making him or her feel different from other children and unwelcome in the classroom. Families are then required to access additional support services at a time when they feel most vulnerable and emotionally depleted.

Accessing Support Services

Often families who are affected by HIV have had to access social service systems all their lives. Most likely they have been confronted with a maze of paperwork and a hostile bureaucracy that has appeared insensitive to their needs. In addition, applying for social assistance can be a very demeaning and demoralizing affair. The eligibility criteria for social programs usually differs from program to program. Understanding the programmatic eligibility differences may be especially difficult for families who have limited education. Families can benefit from guidance in navigating complex social systems.

Services rendered through a case management approach will provide continuity of care and assist the family in the negotiating process. "[Case managers] ensure that children and families have access to all needed services, promote integrated care by linking medical, developmental, and social service providers; follow-up to ensure that families receive the services and that the services are acceptable; advocate for and act as liaisons between the family and other members of the care team; and empower families in the care of their children and themselves."[11] Families coping with HIV may need to be served by many different agencies. A case manager can help provide the coordinated care required, including the initial referral to a hospice program.

Children with AIDS and their families can clearly benefit from hospice services. The multidisciplinary approach to care that hospice brings to families is definitely indicated when caring for a child with AIDS. Families coping with HIV are set apart from all others dealing with a life-threatening illness because of the social stigma associated with AIDS. In addition, AIDS is a disease that can affect many family members, thus posing unique challenges to the hospice worker. Over the course of several months or years a single caregiver may witness the death of an entire family. When working with families with AIDS, it is particularly important to pay attention to the potential for staff burnout. However, despite these differences, families who are living with HIV disease need the same support, empathy, and understanding that all families who are dealing with a dying child both require and deserve. Interventions need to be tailored, taking into consideration the complex psychosocial, environmental, and cultural factors of each family and the vacillating nature of the infection itself.

THE ILLNESS-WELLNESS CONTINUUM

Helping Families Plan for the Future

Despite the unique social challenges facing HIV-infected children and their families, the advances in antiretroviral therapies are permitting children to live longer. One of the most challenging clinical tasks throughout the course of the child's illness is helping families plan realistically for the future. For example, some parents may have questions about how to enhance normal development. Other parents require guidance in enrolling their child in a preschool or school program. Parents may also request information on camp programs, guidance in preparing a preadolescent girl on beginning her menses, of counseling an adolescent about birth control and safer sex practices. Many parents of chronically ill children are relieved to be able to discuss their thoughts regarding resuscitation and life supports. They may feel strongly that they want their child to die at home in his/her own bed. Others may have equally strong feelings against their child dying at home. Many parents are unfamiliar with services such as hospice or home care agencies that provide for pain control and in-home nursing services. Parents often want information about how death may occur, if it will be painful, and how to best comfort their child emotionally and physically during this process. Parents often have questions about funeral costs and procedures, especially in light of some of the "horror stories" about funeral homes not accepting AIDS patients.

Helping Families Plan for the Time of Death

Due to the unpredictable nature of HIV, it is not always possible to plan for the child's final days, weeks, or months but it is useful to help parents feel prepared and in control as much as possible about the events leading to and following the death of their child. It is usually when the child is medically stable that parents find it least frightening to talk about terminal care and to begin thinking about future care needs for the child and family. However, it is often not until a child develops some profound impairment that the full implications of the disease become an emotional reality. This is a good time to help parents explore local resources such as home care or hospice care. It is also a good time for the child to be able to make a wish of his or her own through organizations such as The Make-A-Wish Foundation and Starlight Express.

Parents almost always benefit from guidance about discussing death with their child. In fact, in a recent needs assessment carried out at the Pediatric Branch of the National Cancer Institute, almost one-half of the parents of HIV-infected children reported needing help in learning how to talk to their child or children about death. Parents often worry that if they raise the subject with their child, the child would automatically assume that death was imminent. However, when children are given the opportunity in individual sessions, they frequently talk, write, and draw pictures about their feelings, concerns, and fears about dying. For example, a 6-year-old girl, whose mother was sure she had no idea that she was dying, drew a picture of a rainbow. Around the rainbow she wrote, "This is heaven for when I die." Sharing the drawing with her mother paved the way for open and honest communication between them. Children often have strong images about death or heaven, but because of fear of making their parent(s) anxious, they may keep these images to themselves. Misperceptions and fears can be worked through when the child is provided the opportunity through creative play, art work, or dialogue to express their inner thoughts.

The following stories were written by children during individual therapeutic interviews. Each was asked to complete the paragraph "I Often Wonder. . . . " The content was then used to further explore the child's understanding about what was happening to him or her. With the children's permission, the material produced was also shared with their families. In each case, death and other issues became subjects that could be discussed openly. Children and parents alike cope much better when there is open communication about living as well as expression of their feelings about dying.

> I often wonder what it would be like if I died next month or even sooner. What would happen to my Mom, Dad, and sister after I had gone away. I would miss them alot and I love them so much. I want them to remember me the way I was—happy, loving and handsome.

> I often wonder what heaven is like. I think there are angels all over, baby angels and grown up angels. I also think my friends are there and are happy. When I die I will see them there. I think I too will be happy in heaven.

> I often wonder how often I'm going to get sick and what will happen to me during those times. . . . I often wonder how much longer in life I have. Sometimes I think I only have months to live, other times I'm more hopeful and I think I'll live at least a couple more years. The thought of not living long scares me. Especially dying.

The Child with AIDS: Their Own Death

Children faced with a life-threatening illness often seem to have an intuitive sense about what is happening even before this is discussed with them. However, with HIV this sense is often even more acute. Many HIV-infected children have witnessed the progressive illness and death of one or both parents and often siblings and friends. Due to the stigma associated with AIDS, many HIV-infected children have been asked to lie about their illness. As a result, these children frequently develop an unspoken sense of shame about their disease and about what is happening to their bodies. While a child's awareness and understanding of impending death varies with developmental age, it also depends very much on the social climate that surrounds them during the course of infection and terminal illness. Not only is there a need for open communication between family members and health-care professionals but equally important is the need for trust, acceptance, and physical touch.

Newborn through Toddlers

Children under the age of 2 are not able to conceptualize illness and death and so the trauma of illness falls primarily on their caregivers. Infants and toddlers are most concerned with immediate events (physical trauma) and fear separation from parents and other loved ones. They respond best to a consistent setting, love, reassurance, and being held.

Preschoolers

Preschoolers understand that their disease is not getting better and that they need to take more medicines and spend more time in the hospital. Children this age often engage in play about heaven and "sleeping forever." Such play may be charged with anxiety especially as it relates to the separation from loved ones. Play therapy can help reduce anxiety and better ascertain the child's feelings, concerns, and fears. Consistent parental care, staff, and play areas are useful in helping the child cope with his or her illness. An honest approach to hospitalizations and medical procedures is imperative for preschoolers and school-age children.

School-Age Children

Many parents of HIV-infected school-age children remain ambivalent about informing their child about the true diagnosis because of the potential negative social consequences if the child informs others. However, many of these children are aware of a "secret" in their family. They talk and listen to other HIV-infected children in the hospital setting and, if cognitively unaffected, are generally aware of their serious illness. The need for open communication is essential, especially for those families who have not revealed the true diagnosis. How a school-age child copes with his or her impending death depends greatly on his or her experience throughout the illness. Have they already lost a parent(s) to AIDS? Do their friends know about their infection? Are they still their friends? Have they been allowed to remain in school? Have other HIV-infected children they know died?

Both school-age children and adolescents wonder what will happen to their family once they are gone. They have images of what life will be like for those they leave behind and they benefit greatly from being able to talk about these feelings openly. The following vignette was written by a 14-year-old boy during a clinical interview:

> I worry most about what my dying will do to my family. I want them to be able to go on with their lives and not be depressed all the time. In fact, if I was in Heaven and looking down on my family I would want to see them getting along with each other.

Many older school-age children like to leave drawings, letters, clothes, and other items to those whom they will leave behind. In fact, a few of the children with whom we have worked are in the process of writing a book about their experiences with HIV, in an attempt to educate others. Such a book is an invaluable memoir for the family. Children often enjoy being able to fulfill a wish of their own through organizations such as The Make-A-Wish Foundation. Making a wish allows the child to make decisions about what he or she wants at a time when, in reality, the child has little control over his or her day-to-day life and its finality.

Adolescents

Almost all HIV-infected adolescents are aware of the true nature of their illness and have had to face the fear of (or the reality of) rejection by peers. Adolescents are acutely aware of the finality of death. The kind of experiences they have had, their self-image, and the quality of peer and family relationships will greatly affect their ability to cope throughout the end stages of illness. The particular physical manifestations of disease also play a major role in adolescents' adaptation. The adolescent who "looks" significantly different from his or her peers incurs additional stresses and feelings of loneliness and isolation when they are most in need of support, acceptance, and touch. In fact, direct physical contact by touching and holding, traditional gestures of great comfort, is crucial when anyone is faced with AIDS. It is not only interpreted as a sign of compassion but one of validation that the ill individuals are not pariahs or carriers of disease. Masks, gowns, gloves, and other paraphernalia are very disturbing to all HIV-infected children, and especially to those who are struggling with low self-esteem, guilt, and isolation.

Helping a child to understand death requires insight into the cultural, religious, and philosophical outlook of each family constellation[12] as well as into the fears and images colored by the death of others they have known well. When other HIV-infected children die, the opportunity to ventilate fears, anxiety, sadness, and anger needs to be provided. Children often describe feeling as if they are looking into a mirror. They also often describe not having the chance to say good-bye and wondering when their turn will come. Frequently, we encourage children to write a note to be read at the funeral or to be buried with their friend. The following letter is just one example:

> Dear ____
>
> I miss you very much. But I've learned now that when you're up in heaven that there's no more pain. And last time I saw you, you were in pain. I hope that you are happy now. I will always remember you, because you were such a *good friend*. I love you.
>
> Good Bye,
> Your friend,

The Parents' Perspective

During the final stage when there is a consensus that the end of the child's life is near, the family should be encouraged to decide where the child's final days will be spent. This period often brings confusion to families as they vacillate between wanting to keep their child alive for as long as possible and wanting the child to die with dignity, without pain or discomfort. Enjoying the remaining time with the child needs to be the highest priority during this time. Engaging hospice care is of utmost importance for those parents who wish for their child to remain at home. Parents who are ill may have physical limitations on caring for their child. As much support as possible from family, community, and the health-care team will be needed.

A minority of parents decide to relinquish their children prior to their death due to an inability to care for their child.[13] Special consideration needs to be given to the parents whose child is in care outside of the biological home. Input from the parents on the child's favorite activities, toys, books, foods and security objects as well as inclusion of the parent on discussions of medical treatment can help both the parent and child to be more accepting of decisions that are made, and enable the parent to support the child during visits.[3] Parents also often feel divided at this time between the needs of their dying child and those of the siblings, whose pain is just as real, though invisible.

Siblings

The devastating impact of HIV on siblings is often underestimated. Siblings are emotionally affected from the time of diagnosis and this effect lasts throughout the course of illness and beyond. Siblings of HIV-infected children are not only grieving for the dying child but also for one or both parents who may be ill or have already died. They are often infected themselves and worry about their own deterioration and death. Siblings who are not infected often experience feelings of guilt for being well. They too need an opportunity to express their fears, grief, and thoughts about their sibling without feeling they are further burdening those they love. There are a number of common fears that siblings frequently express including coming home from school and finding a family member gone and of the principal coming to their classroom door to inform them that one of their family members has died. Although siblings routinely endure changes in daily routine due to illness, hospitalizations, and erratic caretaking, they struggle to try to find meaning in a time of emotional chaos, as the following vignette illustrates:

> I think my brother has become a very strong person inside and keeps on getting stronger with every battle against the AIDS virus, he wins. Someday I know he won't be able to win a battle, and he'll go to heaven, but that doesn't mean that he got tired of fighting. I know I'll miss him when he goes, but I also know that he won't hurt anymore.

In fact, many siblings begin developing philosophical views of life and death. The following letter was written during what was believed to be the final hospitalization for this 15-year-old's brother:

It's Hard . . .

It's hard going hour by hour, day by day seeing your brother get weaker and weaker, sicker and sicker.

It's hard knowing that your brother is going to die from a horrible disease like AIDS and you have no control over anything.

It's hard saying good-bye or good night and not knowing if it is the last good-bye or good night that you're going to say to him.

It's hard not knowing where he is going next. But god has good reasons for doing everything that he does and we will just have to learn to except them.

Grandparents

Throughout this epidemic, grandparents have perhaps been among the hardest hit. They are experiencing the potential loss of two generations: their children and their grandchildren. More and more grandmothers are assuming care for their grandchildren following the death of their own child. The impact of the loss of their child is tremendous, their fear of facing death again is great, and, for many, their own health is of concern. A feeling of being overloaded in terms of tasks and responsibilities is a common theme among grandparents. The following quote taken from a support group for grandmothers summarizes the feelings expressed by many:

Everywhere you turn is a problem. As a grandmother you try to be everything to everyone. If you don't, you feel guilty. When you're not able to do it all — because of your own health — you feel guilty too. There just always seems to be the expectation that 'Good ole mom can handle anything'.

No other contemporary disease challenges the integrity of families and results in so many losses as the AIDS epidemic. The following quote illustrates the multiple losses grandparents often face:

Sometimes it's best not to know what will happen next. I don't know what to pray for . . . so many losses . . . I don't really want it to be over. . . . But the gains are so few compared to the losses.

Grandparents need a tremendous amount of support and guidance as they are often not well educated about AIDS. They may not always be present at the hospital or clinic, but their support "behind the scenes" is often the foundation that keeps the family together.

Postdeath

The actual death of the child initiates an extended period of grieving that is both intense and slow to resolve.[14] The death of a child shakes the foundation of the family and it is this loss of a "normal" future that casts doubt on the stability of the family unit.[12] Many parents receive their primary support from the child's health-care staff and from other parents. When the child dies, this routine is aborted and parents experience this as another loss.[13] Regular phone contact between the health-care providers and the family following the child's death allows family members the opportunity to reflect on the child's life and the illness-dying-death experience until acceptance occurs.[15]

Since most parents are HIV-infected themselves, the death of the child raises fears in themselves. Some parents only want to live long enough to care for their sick child. Many parents have other children (infected and noninfected) to care for and are most concerned about how long they will remain well. Although no studies have been completed that assess parental coping following the death of a child with AIDS, in our experience there are several high-risk factors that influence postdeath adaptation. These include the health status of the parent(s) and other family members, the number of losses that have already taken place within the family, whether the parent is a single parent, whether close friends and family are aware of the true diagnosis, the quality of the child's and the family's life prior to the child's death, financial stresses, and the quality of support available during the child's illness and following the child's death. An assessment of the above factors should be made as early in the child's disease as possible so that appropriate supports can be put into place. Many parents maintain ongoing contact with the staff for support throughout their own illness. The death of one's child is an event that is emotionally revisited frequently, and is especially remembered when the parent is facing the same infections, procedures, and events their deceased child only recently experienced.

THE NEED FOR REMEMBRANCE

Parents with AIDS: Terminally Ill Parents with Terminally Ill Children

One of the greatest fears HIV-infected parents face is that of dying before their child. The thought of being unable to protect their child when hurt, comfort their child when sad, and nurture their child when sick is a tragedy almost too painful for parents to consider. Helping parents take an active role in their own health care needs to be a priority. Encouraging parents to make both prospective plans for the child's health care and custody arrangements is also an equally important priority. Assisting parents in identifying future care providers for their children, ensuring a durable power of attorney, and arranging legal custody is best done as early as possible.[13] It affirms parents' control over their family situation and it reassures their children as to who will raise them. If family members or others are not identified, foster care or other alternative care will be needed.

A central theme for many HIV-infected parents is "How will my child(ren) remember me?" This desire to be remembered and the parents' wish to guide their children into the future led to the development of a program that utilized videotapes prepared by parents for their families.[16] These tapes are then left for their children and other family members in the event that the parent dies before his or her infected child(ren). The tapes provide the parent with an opportunity to say good-bye to his or her child and to share many thoughts that the child might be too young to understand at the time of the parent's death or that the parent was reluctant to express face to face. For a child old enough to appreciate such a tape, it may provide added strength to face his or her own disease, the ability to "see" his or her parent when feeling most alone, and also provide a sense of security in knowing the intensity of the parent's love. Properly timing the production of such a tape is essential as parents need to be emotionally prepared to undertake such an important and difficult process and should be in relatively good physical health, as children often refer back to how their parent "looked" on the videotape. For parents who have made such a tape, the taping has been recalled as one of the most significant and intense events throughout the course of their own and their child's infection. Therefore, preparing for the taping requires a delicate balance between fostering hope about their child and family survival without the parent, while maintaining a realistic perspective about the words they want to leave behind and how they want to be remembered. For example, some parents want to film the different places the child and family may have lived (their roots), while others feel more comfortable talking about the cultural beliefs and values by which they wish the child to live. Some parents like to be filmed by themselves, others with their child. It is best for the parent to speak in his or her native language. Because of the emotional intensity, these tapes are best made with the help of a social worker or mental health professional with whom the parent has worked closely.[13,16] For those parents who are not able or comfortable making such a film, other ways to create a feeling of remembrance are needed. For example, creating an album of photographs and stories, leaving special jewelry or clothing for the child to wear, or writing poems or letters have also been extremely useful memories for children.

The Child's Perspective

Understandably, the children often lack ways to express the complex emotions associated with a parent's impending death. If possible, children should be allowed to visit the parent during the illness to permit as much interaction as possible and also to enable the child to gradually develop an awareness that the parent is very sick and that the illness is life-threatening, and to develop some understanding of death as a process, not as an immediate event where the parent disappears out of his or her life.[3] If the dying parent cannot have visitors or the child cannot visit for medical reasons, telephone contact, photographs, handmade "presents," and artwork can help maintain the connection and later serve as concrete items to help the child grieve this loss.[3] Holidays have special meaning to the dying parent and to his or her child. Allowing the parent to plan the child's birthday and any other important holidays helps maintain family harmony at a time of confusion, sadness, and fear of disintegration.

Following the death of a parent, the child needs to grieve at his or her own pace. It is important for the child to have the opportunity to participate in the funeral rites. Visits to the cemetery, viewing photo albums, watching family videos, and sharing memories with those who knew his or her parent well is also of utmost value. However, the process of mourning is never really over. New life experiences may appear at any time that provoke for the child aspects of the relationship with their mother which were not significant at the time of death as the following example illustrates. A 5-year-old girl returned to the clinic for evaluation four months following her mother's death. In all previous visits she cried throughout each blood draw. This visit she did exceptionally well during the procedure but began crying hysterically a few minutes after it was over. She knew her mother would never see how well she had done. She knew her mother would not be able to hold her when she did become very sick.

Following the parent's death, providing the continuity of guidance and support throughout the child's terminal illness can be emotionally rewarding and exceptionally taxing for the staff.

Staff

HIV-infected children are living longer than initially expected and as a result health-care providers become involved in the issues that surround children's lives—school, day care, community programs, and others. Complex clinical, social, and ethical decisions need to be made throughout the course of a child's infection.[17] It is not just the child who is dying, but often the child's HIV-infected parents, brothers, sisters, and extended family members as well. AIDS-related grief becomes cumulative. Staff members do not have the time to absorb the pain and recuperate from multiple losses. Working with people who lives are in continual crisis and with children who are terminally ill requires resilience, stamina, fortitude, strong self-esteem, and creativity as well as a high level of dedication and skill.[1] Staff members require daily team support, good supervision, and consultation. A time for reflection, collaboration, and a feeling of mutual respect is needed. Flexible work schedules have been of great assistance in many settings. Opportunities to work through these important losses are essential, as is respecting the different coping and grieving styles among the health-care team. Some ways that have been helpful have included time to attend the child's funeral, ongoing or as-needed support groups, a memorial garden, and an avenue for staff to remain in contact with family members with whom they had invested much time, love, and effort.

Clearly AIDS will affect the fabric of our society for generations to come. The challenge is to discover ways to effectively treat those individuals who are currently infected and to prevent the infection of individuals at risk. At the same time, it is imperative that the care for children and families with HIV infection not only include attention to the medical needs but also to the dignity of their lives and deaths.

NOTES

1. Lewert, G. (1988). Children and AIDS. Social Casework: The Journal of Contemporary Social Work 69:348–354.

2. Aldape, T. and C.I. Hanson (1990). Pediatric HIV infection and AIDS: A psychosocial perspective. Seminars in Pediatric Infectious Disease 1:170–173.

3. Dubik-Unruh, S. (1989). Children of chaos: Planning for the emotional survival of dying children of dying families. Journal of Palliative Care 5:10–15.

4. Weinberg, D. and H. Murray (1987). Coping with AIDS: The special problems of New York City. Sounding Board. N Engl J Med 317:23.

5. Kübler-Ross, E. (1990). Advocating for AIDS children: A call to action. In G. Anderson (ed.), Courage to Care: Responding to the CRISIS of Children with AIDS. Washington, D.C.: Child Welfare League of America, pp. 295–303.

6. Centers for Disease Control (1991). HIV/AIDS Surveillance Report. Washington, D.C.: U.S. Government Printing Office, February, pp. 1–18.

7. Baker, L. (1992). The perspective of families. In M. Stuber(ed.), Children and AIDS. Washington, D.C.: American Psychiatric Press.

8. Brown, G., J. Mitchell, and S.B. Williams (1992). The African American community. In M. Stuber (ed.), Children and AIDS. Washington, D.C.: American Psychiatric Press.

9. Centers for Disease Control (1989). AIDS Cases Reported Through November 1989. HIV/AIDS Surveillance Report. Atlanta, GA, December.

10. Kübler-Ross, E. AIDS, The Ultimate Challenge. New York, Macmillan, 1987.

11. Family-Centered Comprehensive Care for Children with HIV Infection. Panel on Women, Adolescents and Children with HIV Infection and AIDS. U.S. Department of Health and Human Services, Public Health Service, August 1991.

12. Chanock, S.J., F.L. Johnson, V. Kundra and M.D. Singer. The other side of the bed: What caregivers can learn from listening to patients and their families. In Principles and Practice of Pediatric Oncology, 2nd edition, in press.

13. Wiener, L.S. and A. Septimus (1991). Psychosocial consideration and support for the child and family. In P.A. Pizzo and C. Wilfert (eds.), Pediatric AIDS. The Challenge of HIV Infection in Infants, Children and Adolescents. Baltimore, MD: Williams and Wilkins, pp. 577–594.

14. Howell, D.A. and I.M. Martinson (1989). Management of the terminally ill child. In P.A. Pizzo and D.G. Poplack (eds.), Principles and Practice of Pediatric Oncology. Philadelphia, PA: JB Lippincott, pp. 991–1002.

15. Koch C.B, J. Herman, and M.G. Donaldson (1974). Supportive care of the child with cancer. Semin Oncol 1:81–86.

16. Taylor-Brown, S. and L. S. Wiener (In press). Making videotapes of HIV-infected women for their children. Families in Society.

17. Anderson, G.R. and J. Emery (1990). Present and future challenges in caring for children with HIV and their families. In G. Anderson (ed.), Courage to CARE: Responding to the CRISIS of Children with AIDS. Washington, D.C.: Child Welfare League of America, pp. 305–319.

PART II

Support Systems

6

Family Dynamics

ANDREW R. TARTLER

There are a variety of feelings and issues that impact on a family and child as they decide to help a child die at home or in a facility practicing the art of hospice care. The following is an approach that is practical and deals with realistic problems. Great numbers of families and children have and will benefit from the philosophy of hospice care. For the professionals involved with providing care to these children and families, this information will be helpful and reassuring as you perform your service. This chapter is dedicated to those families who have permitted their child to be part of the hospice experience.

INTRODUCTION

One of the greatest crises a family experiences is the threat of death of one of its members. Studies have shown that in comparison with other types of bereavement, the grief of parents who have lost a child is particularly difficult. The loss of a child interrupts one of the strongest attachment relationships existing between people.[1] After a review of literature concerning parental reactions to the loss of a child, one author concludes that the death of a child makes the family prone to develop short-term or long-term problems in their adaptation to the loss.[1] While there is conflicting evidence concerning the long-term distress of grieving parents, one study found that two years after a child's death parents showed a symptom profile reflecting significantly greater distress than reported by nonbereaved, nonpatient adults.[2] Pediatric hospice care is an opportunity to reduce the negative impact on a family experiencing the loss of a child and to improve the family's adaptation to the loss of a child.

Pediatric hospice care is a philosophy, not a facility. Consequently, hospice care can be provided in a variety of settings. The role of the children's hospice is to care for the physical, emotional, and spiritual needs of the child with a progressive life-threatening illness and the family, helping them to achieve the best possible quality of life.[3] Issues that pediatric hospice programs are able to address include provision of flexible care, support for the entire family, assistance with anxiety over the relief of symptoms, help with the problems of daily living, and continuity of support after the death of a child.[4] Because the focus of service is the family as a unit, the needs of all members can be addressed and supported.

The Family's Decision

Hospice care must be chosen by the child and family, and not imposed by others. While I believe for most children the home is the right place to die, it is not always the choice of the family or the child and that choice must always be respected. There are several reasons that are commonly acknowledged for why families choose a hospice care alternative. Most often is the desire for care in a nonhospital environment where the emphasis is on emotional support, providing time for talking in a relaxed, homelike atmosphere. A second reason is the desire for medical care that has an emphasis on the relief of symptoms rather than active intervention. A third reason is the need for respite care for the family.[4]

Some of the factors that are considered by families for not choosing home-based hospice care are an unwillingness to continue to live in a house where a child has died, complex symptom control problems, the recognition of the needs of the well siblings, and the child's desire for parents to be in a more protective, supportive inpatient environment.[3]

Basic Requirements for Service

There are two basic conditions that are necessary for hospice care to proceed at home. The first condition is met when curative treatment has been modified or discontinued. The second condition is met when most care will be provided by parents and family with health professionals serving as consultants, not primary providers of care. Supporting these requirements is an important assumption that comfort-oriented care can be given at home by parents and family who are emotionally and technically competent to provide it.

Purpose of Hospice Care

The purpose of a children's hospice program is to make it possible for the family to care for the sick child most of the time by ensuring available community services are involved, providing occasional respite care for the child, making home visits and maintaining telephone contact, offering support and help in the place of the family's choosing during the terminal phase, and providing continuous support following the death of the child.[3]

Sources of Care

There are two primary sources of pediatric hospice care, institution-based services or community-based services. Whether or not a family is provided the option of home-based care may depend to some extent on where the child is treated. Institutions that provide their own home care services offer these services to a greater proportion of terminal children than institutions which primarily rely on community agencies.[5] This factor also influences whether or not the family will accept this option. More families accept the home care option when services are provided by the institution than when provided by community agencies.[5] The belief that hospitalization for terminal illness is always the best alternative for a child and family has been invalidated by current research. Families have demonstrated a remarkable ability to care for children at home faced with a wide variety of medical problems.

Referral

Whether or not a family is ever referred to a hospice program depends on several variables. One study has shown that referrals come from a mix of sources. In a group of twenty-five families in a hospice program, 36% were self-referred, 24% by pediatricians, 20% by social workers, and 20% by "others."[4] Even when home care is available, the option is not offered consistently by staff to all the eligible families. The primary reason for a family not to be referred was based on the staff's assessment of the family or patient characteristics to be inappropriate for home care. The problems indicated most frequently are family instability, single parent home, low socioeconomic status, and complicated medical problems. These are institutional biases that need to be addressed. Studies have shown that restrictive criteria based on family characteristics are poor predictors of the family's ability to provide home care.[5] It is possible for a family to provide hospice care for children despite a wide variety of medical problems. Parents, with the support and consultation of the medical staff, need to decide which terminal care option is the best choice for their child and family.

Benefits of Hospice Care

The benefits of hospice care for the quality of life for dying children and their families have been shown in many studies. Generally, the results have demonstrated that patients have a higher level of satisfaction with their care, families are better adjusted, some types of pathological bereavement are prevented, and there are decreased costs to the family.[5] Some of the other benefits that have been noted are the improved quality of individualized personal care, the ability of the family to regain a sense of control over circumstances, and an increased sense of family closeness. Because of the demonstrated benefits, hospice care is becoming an integral part of comprehensive pediatric care for those patients who face death.

MAKING THE DECISION FOR CARE

There are three pathways for helping a child and family make a decision about their preference for care as the child's illness moves to a terminal phase. The process of making this important decision is best accomplished over time with staff assistance. If the family and care providers have the benefit of a long-standing relationship, where trust and friendship can be established prior to the onset of the terminal phase, then they can help the family decide where they would prefer the child to die. The first pathway is through existing staff relationships. The second pathway is developed by early parental training and involvement. Parents and families need time and training to feel competent in the care of an ill child at home. As medical settings become more accepting of planning with, rather than for, patients and families, the process of decision making will continue to improve. Experience has shown that parental competence is best developed from the earliest stages of a child's illness. If parents are encouraged to play an active role in their child's care throughout the disease, it will enhance the ability of the family to feel competent about being able to care for the child in the terminal phase of the illness. The third pathway is to promote the acceptance by the family of home health-care workers early in the disease. This accomplishes several positive steps. Home care providers can establish an early relationship that makes the presence of home care personnel seem like a very natural part of the care plan, an element of care that is naturally extended to the terminal phase of the illness. Home care or hospice staff may also educate families about options for terminal care, not just make a placement or recommendation. There is usually more than one option available for the family to consider.

With the right support, training, and encouragement most parents will express their desire to be more actively involved in and gain control over their child's care. A hospice program serves to strengthen the parents' role and can provide them with a sense of accomplishment and purpose. These approaches will help prepare the family to support the desire of a child to die at home.

Hospice care is, of course, not for every child and family and the decision each family makes must be respected and supported with the best interest of the child being the guiding principle.

THE LAST JOURNEY TOGETHER, FACING DEATH

Preparing for the Transition

The family has now begun to make the decision to accept the final outcome of the disease. The goal in this stage is for the members of the family and health-care team to develop together the best plan to support the patient and family. As the decision is being made by a family to provide hospice care, there are changes that need to be considered by the family and staff. The focus of care is now shifting from the institution to the home or hospice program, the goal changes from cure to pain control, and the care moves from staff to family. Some of these changes are subtle and need to be discussed with the family. Understanding these changes in focus and priority will permit the family and patient to obtain the most benefit from hospice care. For example, for the family to become the experts in how to care for this particular child can be a major change in role. The family now assumes the role of teaching the professional staff how best to care for the patient. The altered medical routines and the decrease in medical tests or procedures all need discussion and understanding. These changes in roles and approaches will need to be understood, practiced, and supported. The relationships between members of the family and members of the staff will deepen as the staff visits in the home.[3] The family is now in their own environment and the staff are the ones accepting their hospitality.

Family Providing Care

One of the most important things that can be accomplished in the transition from hospital to hospice is the educational process that occurs with the family (Table 6.1). The health-care team, from the early stages of the child's illness, needs to teach, involve, and create in the parents a sense of competence in helping provide their child's care throughout the disease. If the educational process is accomplished early, the decision for hospice care will be easier.

Sources of Support

At this point the family is feeling an increased need to identify options for support. Because of the demands on the family, they will need to identify

Table 6.1   How Caregivers Can Enhance Pediatric Hospice Care

1. Question the medical care assumption that we plan for and not with patients and families.
2. Educate, discuss, and promote home-based and hospice care to the health-care team.
3. Encourage the health-care team to teach, involve, and create, in the parents, a sense of competence in helping to provide their child's care throughout the disease.
4. Understand that most parents want to be actively involved in and gain more control over their child's care. It strengthens their role as parent and can provide a sense of accomplishment and purpose.
5. Wait for cues from the family before using the term "hospice care." Home care or community-based care may be more appropriate referrals. Try to educate families about options, not placement.
6. Discuss the hospice concept with families as a viable option; one to be viewed as an extension of hospital care that will not sever established hospital ties or relationships.
7. Use home health-care workers as early as possible in the illness.
8. Locate resources for the family as much in advance of need as possible and facilitate the relationships between family and these resources early.
9. Find resources to lessen or relieve the family's concerns about payment for hospice care. Finances can determine where a patient will be cared for in the end.
10. Respond to all coping mechanisms and emotional reactions by loved ones to the dying process in a nonpathological supportive manner.

all the available options and explore some new ones. Frequently, a family may discount a source of support for some reason. Staff need to help families expand their support base and reconsider any source of support that may have been overlooked. Extended family members, neighbors, church contacts, employers, and school systems all have the potential to provide a variety of supportive ideas and programs. Helping the family develop clear identification of needs or ways others can provide support will also be very helpful in this circumstance.

Staff Support

Several concerns present for the parents who learn their child's life is measured in weeks or months. One of the most common is the need to be reassured that everything possible has been done to help their child. It is imperative that parents feel their child has received the very best of medical care and there is nothing more they or the medical staff can do to treat their child. At this point, parents may want to seek other medical advice, look for treatment in other countries, or consult unconventional healers. Some parents may attempt fad or new remedies made popular by the media. The desire to save their child is natural and normal. The need to hold on to hope is also natural. If a family acts without thought and planning at this stage, their actions could bring additional pain and grief. The health-care team working with the family balance between hoping, facing death realistically, and satisfying their need to know they have done all that can be accomplished to save their child.[6]

Impact on Current Treatment

The family will also have important concerns about the implications of the decision to begin hospice care on their relationship with the treatment team and facility. Usually, that is where the longest and most trusted treatment relationships exist and the family naturally has concern about disrupting those relationships. When the family and the treatment facility have the best interest of the child as their guiding principle and the child wants hospice support for this phase of his life, there is no reason why this decision should negatively affect the established treatment relationships. The family should receive every assurance that the child is welcome to return if circumstances require it or if there is a change in plans for the care of the child. Based on the support and comfort the patient and family have found with their treatment, facility staff will still be available if the decision is to move to hospice care away from the treatment center.

Role of Hope

The dynamic of hope is critical in this transition from curative to comfort care. The concept and use of hope is essential to the family for successful transfer to hospice care. The child and family should be told the truth about what is going on in relation to the illness. This decision to tell the truth, however, does not require the child or family to give up hope. Truthful information is shared in age-appropriate language, stories, or in response to questions raised by the child. Much too often hospice care is viewed as a way to help those for whom there is no longer any hope. Hope is instilled by the way of promise, the key is to help the family and child make the transition from hope for cure to hope for comfort, support, and care for the patient and family. These promises can be made and provided by the hospice team.

Realistic Goals

An approach that has also been helpful in the transition to hospice care has been the ability of the staff and family to work together to establish realistic goals. The stress of caring for a dying child at home can wear family strength and resources very thin over time. It is essential that goals be set that are attainable for the family and child. Often quite simple, but important goals will be established. For example, completion of a school year, distribution of belongings to siblings, or less tangible goals, such as assurance that the family will go on or that a parent will be okay, are examples of common goals that can be accomplished with the support of the hospice team.

Feelings and Emotions

The most difficult area for the family is dealing with the multitude of emotions and feelings that will surface at this stage of the process. Their emotions will range from anxiety, fear, guilt, and anger to concern over the impact the child dying at home may have on the siblings in the family. There is much that the staff can do to resolve these issues. The first task is to separate the issues as they surface. Take concerns one at a time and attempt to resolve or plan for how to resolve each one. This approach will help the family settle emotional issues as they surface. The patient, depending on the age, may also have several fears. Most common childhood fears are fear of the unknown, loneliness, loss of family and friends, self-control, or fear of pain and suffering. These fears of the child are best dealt with by a caring hospice care team, working with the family.

Retaining a Sense of Purpose

During this phase of the illness, the time before death, which may last for a substantial or a short period of time, there are several mechanisms available to help the patient and family retain a sense of purpose. All of these mechanisms are the core elements of a hospice program. The patient can maintain a sense of identity by staying in contact with people who are or have been part of his or her life; for example, having friends or neighbors available to visit routinely with the patient and family. Other goals are to reinforce the child's identity by providing a continuity of their life in the family, or to try and continue patterns or maintain established family behaviors to the degree possible under the circumstances. Each family member should be involved or become part of the care in one way or another.[7] There is always some activity or task any family member can become part of for the patient. Reading stories, playing tape recordings, bringing in the pet for routine visits are but a few of the roles family members can play. The provision of hospice care helps with these issues by providing flexible care and support for all the family members, helps with anxiety over symptoms and their relief, helps with the physical problems of daily living, and provides continuity of support after the death of the child.[4]

Every Child Is Different

How staff and family work with a child in this experience will depend on the child's age and stage of development. Every child and family is different and approaches need to be flexible to meet the individualized needs of a particular child and family. There are many excellent sources of information about age and stage of development and perception of death that are relevant to the explanations provided as questions or issues arise. Children appear to know intuitively about the outcome of their illness and are aware on a spiritual level if they are close to death.[7] Telling the child the truth will cause less confusion and distress then having the child experience the difference between what the child senses and what the adults say and do when trying to hide their grief or protect their child.

The sensitive process of helping a family bring a child home to die is now in place. Now there are new issues and problems for the family and staff to face.

TIME GOES BY SO FAST, THERE IS SO MUCH TO DO!

When the child is home or in a hospice program, the most common issue that families discuss is the feeling that time is going by so fast; that there are so many things they would like or need to do and so little time left to get them all accomplished. Hospice staff can help families develop a basis for establishing priorities for important issues.

Parenting a Dying Child

During the prolonged dying process, whether it be short or long, parents will also be faced with issues about how to parent a dying child. They may have felt comfortable with their parenting skills for well children, but feel poorly prepared to parent a dying child and siblings. Making a morgue out of the house while the child is still alive needs to be avoided. When the patient is overprotected, every desire is met, and all fun and laughter stops, the outcome can be difficult for the survivors. When a more normal routine is followed, when fun, laughter, pleasures, and love are shared, the adversity of illness will be much easier to handle.

Brothers and Sisters

The death of a younger or older sibling has a major impact on children of all ages.[1] Children as young as 1 or 2 years old appear to have the capacity for some forms of grief.[1] There is evidence that the more parents talked with siblings about the dying experience, the fewer problems siblings had after the death.[8] During this time and later parents may feel overwhelmed by the sick child's need for support. This feeling can lead to parents partially rejecting the surviving children. In addition, siblings may experience a lack of parenting because the parents are so preoccupied with their own grief. With the support of hospice the outcome may be greatly improved. A positive family environment with high levels of support results in lower rates of disturbance in children.[9] There are certain goals that parents can accomplish at this point that may prevent impairment in siblings. For example, directing their attention to the siblings' needs, helps parents find better ways to meet the needs of siblings, develops relationships with siblings and the health-care team, helps parents discuss death with siblings, and provides follow-up for siblings.[10] When hospice care is provided, it enhances the possibility for the growth of relationships between the dying child and the parents and siblings. Hospice can also make a family unit stronger by sharing the experience of going through a crisis.

Anticipating Grief

As with previous events, patients and families will experience anticipatory grief during this time. How this grief is engaged by the family is important for the future. The family and patient anticipate the pending death of the child and experience grief before the event. It is necessary to help them resolve each episode of grief as it occurs in order for it to be worked through and set aside. They can grieve over what is lost or given up and proceed to engage more fully in life now. This process is a very important way to assure times of satisfaction and accomplishment as an episode of grief is resolved.

How Will Death Occur?

One of the issues that the family will face is when and how will death most likely occur. There are no certain answers to this question. Studies have indicated that between 2 and 40% of families who attempt home care readmitted their child to a hospital for terminal care.[5] The two factors that seem to be the most critical in preventing rehospitalization are planned visitation by staff (hospice or home care) and thorough symptom and pain management. Even with concerns about how death will occur, hospice care helps provide an opportunity for growth in the parent-child relationship if the parent is open to the communication of the child. In almost all instances, the child will talk about issues if the parent will listen.

Respite Care

The strain of caring for the child at home will begin to be evident at this point. The need for respite care may be greater than ever and can be provided by the hospice team. Hospice can also play a role in providing an element of independence for the patient from the family. Some patients feel anxious or frustrated about their forced dependence on their family and the strain it places on them. Hospice can serve to relieve some of those feelings by providing the family support while providing the patient with a sense of security.

I DON'T WANT TO BE LEFT ALONE

As the patient grows weaker and the days before death grow shorter, issues intensify as the strain and stress of dying at home takes its toll on the family system. However, these moments are also some of the most remembered and sacred memories for the family because the positive outcomes from being at home bring potential benefits to all members of the family.

Saving Strength for Important Events

The patient at this point will start to withdraw, conserving strength and energy for important events or activities. Families frequently observe in the patient a heightened concern about being left alone and increased demands for people to spend time with him or her even when resting. Reassurance by family members that the child will not be left alone is important. This reaction of fear when left alone is normal, but it can place extra pressure on the family to meet this need while continuing the daily functions of family life. Respite care is an important service to consider for the child and family at this point.

Making Plans

There are many ways a family can help a child prepare for death or feel more comfortable about letting go as death draws near. Interest will focus within the family on making plans for the child's death and the funeral arrangements. Every family is different but some level of preparation for these two events is important. Older children and adolescents may have very well-developed ideas about how they want their funeral to be arranged. Sometimes a child will want to make a disposition of important objects to special people or siblings. Some children will want to wear special clothing or have special toys or favorite stuffed animals with them. When a family can make these arrangements with a child, it helps to reassure them that they have done all they can do to comfort their dying child.

Remember Me

Another area that is important to children is the assurance that their family will be alright. The child may have realistic fears or unrealistic fantasies about how the family members will cope with his death. It is important to provide the child with information that will assure him the family members will be sad and miss him, but they will be alright and keep the child as a member of the family through their memories.

How Will Death Occur?

Heightened fears and anxiety about how and when the child will die may also surface again. Most of the time parents are frightened about how the child will die, being concerned about bleeding, suffocation, or about their ability to manage. No one can predict how a child may die but most of the time death comes peacefully. Usually, a child will not have a final outburst of pain or period of intense suffering.[6] Death at home can offer a child the comfort of their own room, pets, friends, brothers and sisters, which means the environment is more relaxed than in a typical hospital setting. In a hospice environment or at home, pain control may in fact be easier because the child is more relaxed and has more activity to help keep their mind off the illness. It has also been suggested that death at home permits families to adjust better after the death when care has been provided as a continuation of family life.[6]

After the Death

Rituals surrounding the death of a child are important and families report feeling supported by performing them. Bathing the child, laying out of the child after death, having the entire family with the child, and spending time with the body in an unhurried manner have all been helpful rituals.[4] Intense feelings in the parents after the death are common and will vary among anger, shock, depression, anxiety, mood disturbance, fears of going crazy, and guilt over what they did or did not do.[1] There are several studies that have reported an unusual incidence and severity of problems in siblings who have experienced a death. Siblings will have reactions that will vary among anger, guilt, sadness, anxiety, separation anxiety, worry about health, and increased clinging behavior.[1] Sibling reactions to the death of a child are starting to be better understood and professionals are paying increased attention to their special needs. Bendor has identified several activities that have potential for preventing the psychosocial impairment of siblings: redirecting parental attention to their needs, helping parents meet their emotional needs, developing supportive relationships between siblings and the health-care team, helping parents discuss death with them and have them attend funerals, have post death follow-ups, and involve community agencies in meeting their emotional and social needs.[10] The more that parents talk with the sibling about the experience of dying, the fewer the problems they have after death.[8] Hospice care establishes an increased opportunity for all of these preventive measures to be in place to help siblings prepare for and cope with the loss of a brother or sister. Older children in the family should not be excluded from a child's death and can take an active role in providing care. Over time, the entire family may develop fewer adjustment problems by being involved in providing hospice care to a dying child.

SEARCH FOR A DEEPER MEANING

Following the death of a child there are new and different challenges that face the family. Few marital and family relationships are unaffected by the loss. Some families experience increased closeness while others feel more distance.[1] One researcher found that about one-fourth to one-third of families who experience the loss of an infant have problems with a lack of communication and the synchrony of the grief reaction.[1] Another found that the impact of a child's life-threatening illness alone can be significant. Approximately 30% of the married couples reported substantial marital problems, 45% of the mothers and 27% of the fathers had psychological difficulties, one-third of the families reported financial difficulties, 64% of the mothers gave up employment after the diagnosis to care for the child, and 40% of school-age siblings had psychological difficulties, emotional, behavioral, or both.[4] Usually mothers have a more intense and longer-lasting reaction than fathers.[1] As indicated previously, hospice care is viewed as one factor that can help mitigate the consequences of a child's death on a family. In one study, 72% of the families felt they had been well supported by a hospice program.[4]

Grief Is Different for Each Person

Each member of the family will grieve in a different way and at a different time. The single most important support provided now is the reassurance that grief in all of its variations is the natural response to loss and is not an abnormal reaction. Follow-up or after care is an important element in the hospice program. The healing of grief is usually a long and slow process. Mothers and fathers seem to grieve in different ways. Mothers reported more sadness, anxiety, sleep disturbance, intrusive thoughts and self-reproach than fathers.[1] Fathers experience a sense of emptiness and failure after their child's death. Fathers also seem to be unwilling to talk about the dead child. Some fathers report feeling an obligation to remain strong to care for and support his wife. The major coping mechanism used by fathers is to keep busy, take on more work, and direct their energy outward.[1]

Even though the impact of a child's death can be severe and prolonged there are things that can help a family cope. Social support through the grief process is usually thought to help resolve adaptation problems. Families need not grieve alone; help and assistance is available from a number of sources. There is some evidence that other parents or couples who have lost children are a preferred source of support.[1]

A Deeper Meaning

There are also families who report a more positive outcome from the death of a child. They may begin by looking for a deeper meaning or fuller understanding of their loss. Families may experience a permanent change in their values. For example, they may become more caring toward others or grow to love and appreciate their other children more than before. Some parents may feel they have improved as parents for their surviving children. Siblings may also experience some positive outcomes from this experience. Some report an increased sense of maturity, an improved ability to cope with stress, and an increased empathy with parents. Although the period of grief may be prolonged, with support and help the outcome may be positive for many of the families who experience the loss of a child.

A Member of the Family, Always

The deceased child will always remain a part of the family unit. Parents who have lost a child report an uneasiness in answering questions about how many children they have in their family. The healthiest answer is to always include the deceased child. The memories of and the psychological effects from losing that child are and will continue to be an active part of the family's life.

Those memories of a dead child will be enhanced by providing hospice service to the great number of families who can benefit from the philosophy of hospice care.

SUMMARY

For most children and families home is the right place to die if enough support can be provided. The role of the children's hospice is to care for the physical, emotional, and spiritual needs of the child and family, helping them to experience the best possible quality of life. There are multiple potential benefits available for all members of the family when hospice care is provided. Hospice care is important because it gives families and patients an opportunity to take an active role in the decision-making process about when, where, and how care is provided. The hospice concept is a structured way to provide parents the important opportunity to parent and meet the needs of their dying child while continuing to meet the needs of other family members. Even at this time of anguish, hospice enhances this chance for the family to gain strength, closeness, and maturity.

NOTES

1. Dyregrov, A. (1990). Parental reactions to the loss of an infant child: A review. Scand J Psychol 31:266–280.

2. Moore, I.M., C.L. Gilliss, and I. Martinson (1988). Psychosomatic symptoms in parents 2 years after the death of a child with cancer. Nursing Research 37:104–107.

3. Dominica, Mother Frances (1987). The role of the hospice for the dying child. Br J Hospital Medicine, October:334–343.

4. Stein, A., G.C. Forrest, H. Woodley, and J.D. Baum (1989). Life-threatening illness and hospice care. Arch Dis Child 64:697–702.

5. Lauer, M.E., R.K. Mulhern, R.G. Hoffmann, and B.M. Camitta (1986). Utilization of hospice/home care in pediatric oncology: A national survey. Cancer Nursing 9:102–107.

6. Adams, D.W. and E.J. Deveau (1984). Coping with childhood cancer, where do we go from here? Reston, VA: Reston Publishing Company.

7. Kübler-Ross, E. (1983). On children and death. New York: Macmillan.

8. Birenbaum, L.K. (1989). The relationship between parent-sibling communication and coping of siblings with death experience. J Pediatr Oncol Nursing 6:86–91.

9. Keitner, G.L. and I.W. Miller (1990). Family functioning and major depression: An overview. Am J Psychiatry 147:1128–1137.

10. Bendor, S.J. (1990). Anxiety and isolation in siblings of pediatric cancer patients: The need for prevention. Social Work in Health Care 14:17–35.

7

Caring for Bereaved Parents

J. WILLIAM WORDEN and JAMES R. MONAHAN

The death of one's child can be one of the most difficult losses to grieve. This is especially true when the child is underage and still considered a child. There are a number of factors that contribute to this difficulty. Hospice care personnel need to understand these factors, to know what the issues are for bereaved parents, and to know how to intervene with appropriate and facilitating interventions.

This chapter examines (1) stresses on the parent, couple, and family after the death of a child; (2) risk factors for poor outcome; and (3) goals and strategies for intervention with bereaved parents.

STRESS ON THE PARENT

There are a number of factors that influence the stress experienced by a bereaved parent. The most obvious is the untimeliness of the death. Parents are supposed to outlive their children, and the death of a child flaunts this natural order. This "out-of-season" death challenges the parent's need to find some meaning in the death. Frequently asked questions are Why me? Why my child? Where was God? How can I go on? Such meaning is not easy to find and can challenge the parent's belief system about the world and provide a major spiritual crisis. Quite often bereaved parents report changes in fundamental life values and philosophical beliefs as a consequence of experiencing the death of a child.[1]

It is the role of parents to protect their children, especially underage children. The death of the child assaults this role and is one of the major stressors when a child dies. How could I have not prevented this from happening?

Guilt is a frequent feature of bereavement and this is especially true for bereaved parents. Miles and Demi have posited five types of guilt that bereaved parents may experience.[2] The first is *cultural guilt*. Society expects parents to be guardians of their children and to take care of them. The death of one's child is an affront to this social expectation and may lead to this type of guilt. *Causal guilt* is a second type. If the parent was responsible for the death of the child through some real or perceived negligence, the parent may experience causal guilt. Causal guilt can also be a part of the parent's experience when the death occurs from some inherited disorder. *Moral guilt* is characterized by the parent feeling that the death of the child was due to some moral infraction in their present or earlier life experience. There is a variety to such presumed infractions. One frequently seen is residual guilt from an earlier terminated pregnancy. Because I elected to terminate a pregnancy, I am now being punished for that act by losing my child. *Survival guilt* may also be found among bereaved parents. Why did my child die and I am still alive? Survival guilt is more frequently found when the parent and child have been involved in the same accident and the parent survives when the child does not. Finally, there is *recovery guilt*. Some parents feel guilty when they move through their grief and want to get on with their lives. They believe that such a recovery somehow dishonors the memory of their dead child and that society may judge them negatively.

Bereaved parents often have the need to blame someone for the death of their child. Such a need is strong when the child died in an accident or by suicide or homicide. But the same can hold true when the child dies of natural causes. Sometimes this need to blame is targeted toward a marriage partner or other family member and places stress on the family system. It is also possible for a family member, such as a child, to be scapegoated after a death. Counselors need to be aware of these dynamics and help a family to find an appropriate place for their anger and their blame.

Concurrent losses after a child's death can also lead to parental stress. One mother cared for her leukemic child over several years and when he was one of the first to receive bone marrow transplants. After her son died, she became aware that she had not only lost a son but had lost her role as mother of a sick child, something that helped her define herself and provided her with activity to fill the day.

STRESS ON THE MARRIAGE

Incompatible Grieving Styles

Partners do not always have similar styles of expressing grief. This can be due to differences in personality, perceived gender roles, or levels of personal or spiritual development.

Each parent needs to understand his or her own way of expressing grief as well as their partner's grieving style. One partner may be more facile than the other at expressing and discussing emotions. An open expression of feelings may intimidate the other partner, close that partner off to communication, and thus drive the parents further away from each other. When a counselor is working with a couple, it is important not to appear to be siding with the more emotionally expressive partner. If this happens, the less expressive parent may feel left out and become frustrated with the counseling process. At the onset of counseling, the couple's communication with each other may be through the counselor. One parent may reluctantly attend the counseling sessions or go "just to help the other." Often this will be the father. Some people believe that it does not help to dwell on the past, especially the painful past. For this reason they will not speak of the grief they are experiencing.

If partners do not understand each other's ways of grieving, the incompatibility can serve to drive them apart from each other. This can be lonely for the individuals and destructive to the relationship. It happens at the time they need each other the most, when they are feeling the pain of their common loss.

Individual and Gender Differences

Bereaved parents handle grief as they do other major stressors in life. They experience and display grief in a manner congruent with their personality. Most individuals tend to be more introverted or extroverted, more cognitive or emotional. Grief will be experienced and displayed according to these differences.

Extroverts find comfort in being around a group. The group may consist of other grieving individuals or any group of people. An extrovert will want to talk about the loss and ensuing feelings. He or she will probably feel a need to discuss the events leading up to the death, at the time of death, and since the death.

Introverts, on the other hand, usually want to be alone or with a few trusted friends. The introvert has a tendency to internally reflect on the loss and ensuing feelings. If the introvert does discuss the situation, it is more likely to be about conclusions rather than the details leading to these conclusions.

There are also gender differences that play out in the expression of grief. These gender role expectations are part of the socialization process in our society and culture. Studies of men reveal that men are more likely to fear the consequences of emotional expression in a social context. Men disclose far less with less intimate information to others than do women. For men, close friendships are based on shared activities rather than intimacy and assumed loyalties rather than shared feelings. Bereaved fathers are faced with several double binds as they struggle to cope with their child's death. First, fathers are given little social support while they are expected to be a major source of support for their wives, children, and other family members. Second, fathers are confronted with the culturally idealized notion that grief is best handled through expressiveness, while at the same time they need to control such frightening and overwhelming expressions of grief.[3] These conflicts between social and personal expectations can lead men to feel frustration, anger, and aloneness in their grief.

It may be necessary to have a third person, such as a counselor, help the couple understand their individual differences and that there is no correct way to grieve. It is beneficial for each partner if he or she grieves in a style that is congruent with his or her personality and feels understood by the other.

Sexual Intimacy

The death of a child can place strain on a couple's sexual intimacy. Sexual abstinence is frequently reported by couples due to a lack of sexual interest because of overwhelming grief. This lack of interest may be true for one partner but not the other. If so, this will place strain on the relationship.

The opposite can also be true. Sexual activity may be sought out by some couples shortly after the death. For these couples, sexual intimacy serves as a reaffirmation of life and supports their strong need to be close to each other and take care of each other. Johnson studied bereaved couples and noted that some men who previously could not be close to their wives without sexual activity could, after the loss, be close without sex.[4] This change was a surprise to some of the men who now understood why their wives enjoyed and were comforted by hugging.

Divorce Potential

It is important for grieving parents to understand the potential for their relationship to disintegrate. Such parents are frequently reminded by well-meaning friends and family that many marriages end in divorce after the death of a child. If so, this may become a concern of the grieving parents. Data are available that both supports and does not support the break-up of a marriage after the death of a child.

The Society of Compassionate Friends conducted a literature survey and found that, to date, there were no conclusive studies that showed an increased divorce rate resulting directly from parental grief. The results indicated, however, that there was sufficient anecdotal evidence to suggest an increased divorce rate among this population.[5] In the same article, Klass gives an excellent description of the paradoxical effect of the death of a child on the relationship of the parents:

> The shared loss creates a new and very profound tie between them at the same time that the individual loss each of them feels creates an estrangement in the relationship. The paradox is expressed differently in couples with different relationships prior to the death. (p. 239)

Klass summarizes by indicating that the divorce rate may indeed be higher but the increase in the divorce rate may not be a direct result of the death of the child but due to preexisting factors.

If grieving parents are told or read about the increased potential for divorce, it may become the expected outcome. After all, the unthinkable happened with the death of the child, so why not this! A few months after the death of his young son, one father stated, "I am glad that we found out that not all grieving parents get a divorce. I am relieved to know that this does not have to be down the road for us."

The focus of grief counseling should not be on divorce statistics but on surmounting the stressors brought about by the child's death and on addressing underlying marital difficulties.

For some couples, mutual support and intimacy may increase during the intense pain of grief. The opportunity exists for the parents to develop or enhance a supportive relationship and the risks of the situation should be reframed into opportunities to nurture the marriage.

STRESS ON THE FAMILY

Replacement Child

One area of concern for the family and grief counselor is that of the "replacement child." This term refers to the substitution of another child for the child who has died. The replacement child may be conceived subsequent to the death or during the terminal phase of the child's illness. The replacement child could also be an adopted child or a sibling of the child who died. This replacement child is often seen as a second chance or as a way to make up for mistakes or shortcomings the parent(s) perceive in their parenting of the deceased child.

Parents should be encouraged not to have further children until they have worked through the loss of the first child. Otherwise, they may not do the necessary grief work, or they may work out their grief issues on the replacement child.

The child who is placed in this role is also at a distinct disadvantage. Being a replacement child can interfere with cognitive and emotional development. It may lead to a relative absence of the sense of individuality as the child is treated as the deceased sibling.[6] The development of the replacement child is further complicated because replacement children are often overprotected by fearful parents and raised in homes dominated by images of the dead child.[7,8] Replacement children are expected to emulate the deceased child—a child that can be easily overidealized—and are not allowed to develop their own identity.

Roles Played by the Dead Child

Children play various roles in the lives of the parents. After the death, the loss of these roles is accompanied by grief as the parents confront life without each intra- and interpersonal facet added by the child.

Among the various roles a child may play include a sense of intergenerational continuity, a means for the parents to accomplish something that they personally might have been unable to do, a sense of accomplishment, a state of excitement, and something to brighten the day. The child is often the means to starting a conversation with strangers, a source of recognition as strangers pass the parent with a cute baby or child. This attention is often accompanied by a sense of accomplishment and pride by the parent. Whatever the role, these are lost.

The sick or terminal child may have brought about certain recognition. Being a parent of a deceased child places the parents in a new role. The disclosure, by parents, that a child is dying or has died is often met with compassion, sorrow, anxiety, apprehension, or pity. The child continues to play a part in the life and identity of the parent.

Klass asserts that the loss of a child is a permanent condition.[9] It is a loss to the self-image of the parent. He states that the parents face two tasks: (1) learning to live without the child which includes a new form of interacting with the social network, and (2) internalizing an inner representation of the child that brings comfort.

Unaddressed Grief

Some bereaved families have a "no talk" rule and choose to deal with their grief by not addressing it. The deceased child's name may seldom be mentioned. If there are other children in the family, they may not be given full or even factual details of the circumstances surrounding the death. The intention is to protect the siblings from pain or because it is believed that they cannot understand or feel the loss. This situation may arise when the perceived role of the parents is to be strong and strong means showing no painful emotions. Unaddressed grief may also reflect the religious convictions the family hold, namely, that it is wrong to display or feel anything that may convey a doubt in the actions of God. Anger, doubt, or questioning the loss is to question the ways of God.

The absence of discussion of the death or not displaying grief responses leaves the siblings without a model to deal with what they may be feeling or thinking. This "no talk" rule may lead to future problems including an exaggerated fear of death or any objects, events, or people associated with the death. In time this can lead to a delayed grief reaction that may be triggered by another loss years later. The surviving family members may develop an inability to form intimate relationships because of an underlying fear of being abandoned.

It is important for the professional working with such a family to be aware of the "no talk" rule. The professional may point out how important it is for the siblings to learn to express their grief and the potential long-term consequences of unexpressed grief.

RISK FACTORS FOR POOR OUTCOME

Spinetta and colleagues followed bereaved parents for three years after the loss.[10] Parents who were doing better at that time (1) had a consistent philosophy of life that helped them find some meaning in the loss, (2) had viable and ongoing support, and (3) could give their dying child information and emotional support consonant with the child's needs. Parents lacking the above coping mechanisms did less well. One would surmise that parents whose children had longer illnesses would be doing better after the death. Such was not the case, although there was a trend in this direction.

Lack of Support

Grieving is a social phenomenon. For grief to progress and the tasks of mourning to be accomplished, it is important for grieving persons to have the opportunity to express and share their grief with others and to talk about what they are going through. Such sharing includes talk about the events leading up to the death, including the diagnosis, treatment, interaction with others and with the deceased. Some people feel uncomfortable when they are around bereaved parents and may cut off conversations about the deceased. Because of this, support groups for bereaved parents, such as those sponsored by the Society of Compassionate Friends, can be a safe haven for bereaved parents to share their thoughts and feelings with others who have also lost a child.

Segal and associates asked a group of bereaved parents what they would have wanted after the death of their child.[11] Many parents felt that they were given insufficient information. It would have been helpful to have more information as to the cause of death, more information regarding risks to their other children, and information on grief.

When asked to give advice to those who are confronted with grieving parents, the following guidelines were important:

- Take the initiative to contact the parents.
- Don't judge their grief reactions, instead listen to them.
- Give practical help.
- Repeat information as needed; the stress of the situation may preclude one from grasping it the first time.
- Don't offer platitudes or artificial consolation.

INTERVENTION GOALS

Before Death

Bereavement interventions begin before the death of the child. There are several goals for such interventions that hospice personnel need to be aware of. Specific techniques of intervention can be tailored around these goals, depending on the child, the family, and the type of hospice setting and program. Here are some of the important goals.

First, help the family to stay connected with their child until death. For most families this is not difficult and needs little prompting. For others, however, seeing their child declining is a painful situation, and they may have trouble staying connected with the child until the end. One of our clients had a son who was born with major congenital defects. He lived for six years, but during this time he was very demanding and difficult for the mother to manage. During his final hospitalization, she was not there with him and later developed serious clinical depression related to her guilt feelings of abandoning him during this period. It took considerable therapy after the death to help her work through her feelings.

Second, help to facilitate communication. This involves communication not only between the family and the caregiving staff, but also among family members themselves. Being sensitive to what a parent or the patient wants to know or does not want to know is important and faciliating this is a part of good hospice care. Helping parents to say to their child what they need to say before the child dies is important and may preclude regrets after the death.

Third, help the family to develop memories that they can hold and cherish long after the death. Pictures of the child and other family members can be important. Some hospice programs help families to make video tapes of the dying child with other family members. Making these films available to families gives them something concrete that they will cherish and replay over the years as they appropriately memorialize the child in their lives and their family.

Fourth, help parents to negotiate the medical system. Some parents are well skilled in this and do not need our help. Others are more intimidated by the system and are hesitant to ask questions or to assert their preferences. Helping parents to develop these skills through role playing and providing them the encouragement to do what they need to do can be an important part of prebereavement counseling.

Fifth, provide respite care. The demands of caring for a sick child are many and often fall on the shoulders of the mother. The closer to death the child is, the more the mother may want to be with the child. Hospice volunteers are often good resources for this type of respite care so the parent may take a break from their caregiving responsibilities.

Sixth, help parents with the concept of appropriate death. This is a concept developed by Drs. Avery Weisman and William Worden in Project Omega at the Massachusetts General Hospital. An appropriate death is a death that is consonant with the goals, values, and life-style of the individual. Although used more with adults, it can be a useful concept to use with children, particularly adolescents. One late adolescent girl wanted to spend her final weeks of life out of the family home and to be in an apartment near the shore. Although her parents would have preferred to have her at home, they helped her to find such living quarters where she could experience a degree of autonomy, express the individuation appropriate to her age, and to be with her friends—all values that were important to her.

Seventh, prethinking the funeral can be important for some parents. Helping parents to talk about choices and to think of the funeral or memorial service is difficult, but it can also help them plan a service that reflects the uniqueness of the child who is dying. In our experience, including family members such as siblings in the planning can be a worthwhile activity. For some parents, this activity may not be acceptable as it connotes to them a loss of hope and the reality that their child will not make it. However, those parents whose children are under hospice care tend to be more open to planning a service in advance of the death.

After Death

After death, the goals of intervention center around the Tasks of Mourning.[12] Here bereavement is not seen as falling into neat stages or even into predictable phases. Rather, the course of mourning can be seen as involving four tasks that need to be accomplished. These tasks do not need to fall into a specified progression and they can be reworked at various times, depending on the needs of the parents.

The first task of mourning is *accepting the reality of the loss*. Even in the case of an anticipated death, there is a certain sense of unreality after the loved one is gone. This sense of unreality is greatly heightened in the circumstance of a sudden death such as an accident, homicide, or suicide. This acceptance of the reality is not just one of mental assent but involves emotional acceptance as well. One mother, whose 12-year-old daughter was killed in a house fire, went to visit her daughter's grave every day but would not let herself believe that her daughter was dead. For two years she went about saying, "I don't want you dead, I won't have you dead." She finally realized that she was not moving through bereavement and sought out grief therapy. The focus of the therapy involved accepting the reality of her daughter's death, that the daughter would never return, and being able to say good-bye to her.

There are several ways to facilitate this task. If the parents see the body of their child and are able to have a service that commemorates the uniqueness of the child, it will help to bring home the reality of the loss. Talking about the child with the parents, using the past tense, for example, "she was . . . ," and using difficult words like "dead" can be facilitating interactions with bereaved parents. It is also useful to encourage parents to visit the cemetery or other place of final disposition as a part of their grief work.

One of the most difficult things for most bereaved parents to do is to dismantle the room that had belonged to their child and to do something with the child's belongings. There is no set time frame for this difficult task, but at some time it needs to be done. There are some parents who never accomplish this and set up the room as a shrine to the dead child. This avoidance is not a healthy accommodation to the loss. Hearing from the bereavement counselor, "When you are ready, you will," can be a facilitating comment to parents struggling with this decision.

The second task of mourning is *processing the pain of the loss*. This pain involves the strong feelings and sensations that are associated with grief. If these feelings are cut off or not allowed to find an expression, they will remain with the person to be expressed at a later time when a subsequent loss triggers them. Unexpressed feelings can manifest themselves in some type of somatic expression with or without the possible development of some type of illness. The expression of grief comes in many forms and is determined by one's culture, personality, ego development, and the availability of social support. The support of others is most important in order that the person not be overwhelmed by their pain.[13]

Hospice personnel who work with the bereaved can help mourners identify how they are feeling, sanction those feelings that the person may experience as awkward, and help them to find expression of these feelings in a manner that will bring about both relief and resolution.

Several feelings can be problematic for bereaved parents. One of these is anger. Most bereaved parents have some anger, which may include anger at their child for dying and causing them to hurt so much. Displacing this anger onto another person needs to be evaluated by the counselor for its appropriateness and the parent helped to find an expression of this anger that will bring it to conclusion. A father whose teenage son was killed in an automobile accident was not angry with the boy who was driving the automobile at the time of the accident but discovered that he was really angry at the driver's father. Once he discovered this target, he was encouraged to write a letter to the boy's father expressing his strong feelings and to identify the wants he had associated with these feelings.

Guilt is another feature frequently found among bereaved parents. Sources of guilt have been described earlier in this chapter in the section "Stress on the Parent." Some of this guilt is irrational but may resolve after reality testing. Parents who feel that they did not do enough for the child may relinquish this guilt when led to examine just what they did and did not do. Where the culpability is real, parents may need some professional assistance to deal with this.

The third task of mourning is *adjusting to an environment where the deceased is missing.* Some of these adjustments are obvious and others are subtle. An early confrontation for most bereaved parents is how to answer when asked the question "How many children do you have?" The first Christmas brings the dilemma "How many stockings to hang?" Parents try different solutions to these challenges and may change their response as time passes and grief changes.

What one adjusts to depends on the roles and type of relationship that the dead person played in one's life. Children play different roles in the family system and have specific personal meanings for each of the family members. Adjustment takes time, and this is one of the reasons why bereavement can be such a long process. Groups for bereaved parents can be useful, not just for the emotional support they provide, but also because they can be a valuable resource for parents while they are dealing with this third task of mourning.

One dimension of this third task for many parents is finding some kind of meaning from the death of their child. There are various ways parents may go about this. Some find meaning in adherence to religious and philosophical beliefs. Others find meaning through identification of the child's uniqueness and by finding some appropriate memorialization for the child. Still others find meaning by becoming involved in activities that can help individuals and society.[14] Klass found that parents who could transform the parental role of helping and nurturing one's child to helping and nurturing others in a self-help group had more positive and less stressful memories of the deceased child.[9]

The fourth task of mourning is *to emotionally relocate the deceased so that one can move on with life*. Traditionally, the final task of grief has been thought of as withdrawing emotional energy from the deceased and reinvesting it in another relationship.[12] However, bereaved parents have difficulty understanding the notion of emotional withdrawal. How can one ever move away from the attachment that one has to one's child? A more appropriate way to look at this task is one of relocation. The bereaved parent goes through a period of evolution in relation to the thoughts and memories associated with the child, but does this in a way that allows them to continue on with life after the loss.[12] Another way to address this is to think of finding a place in one's life for what one lost—an appropriate memorialization of the deceased.

One parent eventually found an effective place for the thoughts and memories of her dead son so she could begin reinvesting back into life. She said:

> Only recently have I begun to take notice of things in life that are still open to me, you know, things that can bring me pleasure. I know that I will continue to grieve for Robbie for the rest of my life and that I will keep his loving memory alive. But life goes on, and like it or not, I am a part of it. Lately, there have been times when I notice how well I seem to be doing on some project at home or even taking part in some activity with friends.

Here is a bereaved parent who is moving through her grief and carrying on with her life without feeling that she is dishonoring the memory of her child. This goal is the ultimate and the most challenging for any bereaved parent.

INTERVENTION MODELS AND STRATEGIES

There are different models for providing bereavement services to grieving parents. These include (1) individual grief counseling for one or both parents, (2) couples counseling, (3) family counseling, (4) bereavement support groups, and (5) social support groups. The modality of the approach is determined by the request of the grieving parents and the clinical judgment of the counselor. Alexy found that bereaved parents wanted different kinds of counseling depending on which phase of mourning they were in.[15] Murphy and colleagues found that the timing of the intervention was as important as the intervention itself, when measuring the effectiveness of bereavement intervention.[16]

Individual Grief Counseling

The goal of grief counseling is to assist the grieving person with the various tasks of grief. Videka-Sherman pointed out that the adaptive task of grief counseling is not to change the reality of the loss, but to help parents adjust to the reality.[17] Grief counseling assists the client with this task. Counseling is often helpful when the individual feels frustrated or stuck in the grief process. Because normal grief can take on so many forms, individuals may feel as if they are not grieving appropriately or for the correct amount of time. The belief that the grief process is not following a "correct" course may be supported by well-meaning family members and friends. They often tell the grieving person that there must be something wrong because the intensity, variety, and duration of symptoms should be subsiding and the parent should be getting on with life. The first six months is often the time when grieving parents seek counseling because they are hurting and receiving messages that the pain is abnormal.

Couples Grief Counseling

Couples counseling is appropriate when grieving couples are in need of help with their communication skills. Communication may be deficient for a number of reasons. Causes of incomplete communication include (1) single focus communication when the child was ill. Because the focus for each parent may have been on the needs of the child, there may not have been much demand for communication other than about the child; (2) one parent is protective of the other. When one parent is feeling especially pained and the other appears to be having a good day, the hurting partner does not want to ruin the seemingly positive mood of the other; (3) one parent may misinterpret the behavior of the other because of different grieving styles; (4) the child may have kept the couple together. After the child is gone, the reason for staying together is also gone. However, leaving and facing another loss at this time may be unbearable so the couple stays together physically but not emotionally; (5) one parent may believe that it is a sign of weakness to discuss or display painful emotion to the other; (6) there may be anger or guilt about the death that is displaced or projected onto the other spouse. The counselor's role is to help identify the issues behind poor communication and to facilitate more effective interactions.

Family Counseling

The goal of family grief counseling is to assist the family to adapt to life without the deceased child. The family is an interactive system. When one part of the system is changed or removed, the whole system is affected. The death of a child challenges the systemic balance of the family.

The child who died played various roles in the family and had different relationships with surviving family members. Each family member will grieve differently because each has had a unique relationship with the deceased and must embark on a personal odyssey through the mourning process and confront what he or she has lost.[18]

Also, the deceased child performed many tasks within the family. The replacement for each of these tasks will have to be addressed as they arise. These tasks may be concrete,such as doing household chores, or they may be abstract, such as being the son we wanted and finally had.

The grief of grandparents is also a part of the family picture though it is sometimes overlooked. Often grandparents experience anger and disappointment over the child's illness and death and may point the finger of blame onto the parents. Occasionally, these blame scenarios are switched when the mother of a dying child is disappointed in her own mother's inability to understand and to offer emotional assistance.

It is important that the needs of the siblings be addressed as well as those of the parents and grandparents. The surviving siblings may feel left out as a result of the attention that is or was being paid to the terminally ill or deceased brother or sister. Siblings may have been told, or otherwise perceived, that their own needs came after those of the child who is dying. Unless this belief is changed, it could have long-lasting effects on the sibling's self-esteem.

Surviving brothers and sisters may also experience guilt. The etiology of this guilt is as varied as the personality and developmental level of the sibling. It may be due to a sense of relief at the death because their own needs were overlooked in favor of those of the deceased. Guilt may also arise as a result of sibling rivalries or arguments prior to the illness and death. There may be a form of survivor guilt if the dead sibling was treated as a very special child and received more attention than the surviving brother or sister. This guilt could lead to the belief that the deceased was more worthy of life and the wrong child died.

Magical thinking may also play a part in the grieving process of younger children. Magical thinking is the belief held by children that they somehow caused or helped bring about the death by their thoughts or unrelated actions prior to the death. Magical thinking may also be present after the death. A child may believe that the deceased may be brought back by strong wishing or even by certain behaviors.

Unspoken family rules are often established to dictate if, how, and when grief may be expressed. But feelings that are not expressed do not vanish. They become part of the underlying system that governs individual choices and behaviors. In order for the family to successfully adjust to life without the lost child, the new family circumstances must be investigated and discussed.

Virginia Satir describes the ghosts that may be part of a family system.[19]

> I believe that anyone who has ever been part of a family system leaves a definite impact. A departed person is often very much alive in the memories of those left behind. . . . If the departure has not been accepted, for whatever reason, the ghost is still very much around and can disrupt the current scene. (p. 185)

The manner in which children grieve is often learned from their parents. Children of parents who do not express emotions will tend to be unexpressive. Often, children are excluded from discussion or information about grief or the dying and death of the sibling. This may be done in an attempt to protect the surviving children from the pain of the grief. Whatever the reason, this protection may make it more difficult for the child to grieve. Accurate information is vital to the successful resolution of the grief process. Children do not have the same opportunity to gather information or seek a sympathetic person as do adults. Usually the only source of information and sympathy for the child is the family.[20] If information is not forthcoming, the child might imagine circumstances to fill in the void. This may be worse than reality. Family grief counseling should include information and education for the parents in order that they might assist the surviving children with their grief. As children mature and develop, they need to reprocess the loss. It is important that the parents continue to provide support and information to them.

Bereavement Support Groups

Individuals who are reluctant to seek individual, couple, or family counseling may be more inclined to attend a bereavement support group. Support groups may seem less intimidating than counseling or therapy and are more likely to appeal to a wider range of people.

There are a number of approaches that may be taken when planning a bereavement support group. These depend on the needs of the population and the personnel available to conduct the groups. Groups may be on-going or closed-end. They may meet once a week, for six or eight weeks, once a month, or indefinitely. They may include a specified topic of discussion, a presentation, or whatever the group decides on. They may be closed or open to new participants. These groups may include social functions or be limited to grief-related discussion. They may be any combination of the above. It is important to be flexible and try different approaches in order to meet the needs of those attending.

The following topics are appropriate for bereavement support groups: symptoms of normal grief, changing roles/changing identities, guilt and anger, stress management, and getting through the holidays. Other topics specific to parental grief may be discussed such as parenting the surviving children while grieving, helping the other children with their grief, examining spiritual issues that arise as the result of surviving one's child, and having other children.

The most beneficial component of a support group is contact with others who have a clear understanding of what one is experiencing. To hear the stories of others who are experiencing the same symptoms is often reassuring to the grieving parents. When parents learn that they are not the only ones to experience the unique painful reactions of parental grief, there is less of a tendency to judge their reactions as abnormal. This participation can reduce the anxiety and fear that accompanies new painful experiences and lead to increased feelings of relief and normalcy.

Videka-Sherman and Lieberman looked at the effects of participation in self-help groups by bereaved parents.[21] They found that such participation changed the parents' attitudes about bereavement but did not have a major impact on the parents' mental health or on the marital functioning of the couple.

Social Support Groups

These groups are a very important aspect of bereavement services. Social get-togethers, such as luncheons, pot-luck suppers, picnics, and other outings, provide a means for bereaved parents to meet each other. These settings are not perceived to be as threatening as support groups or counseling sessions. Although social get-togethers are not therapy sessions, they can be therapeutic. Parents meet others who have experienced similar losses, hear about coping techniques, and may feel less anguish because they are no longer the only ones they know who have suffered such a tragedy.

Social support groups provide an excellent opportunity for grieving parents to "compare notes" and normalize painful experiences. At one get-together at a popular restaurant, one of the bereaved asked another how she felt when she saw the deceased in the coffin for the first time. This is not the usual luncheon chatter, but it was important for the two to share their perceptions, feelings, and thoughts about this very difficult experience.

CONCLUSION

The death of a child is one of the most difficult losses to grieve. The losses continue to present themselves long after the pain of other deaths might have subsided. Graduations, marriages, births, children playing, or any other event can serve as a reminder for what might have been, if the child had survived, and bring about renewed pain.

One grieving mother said, "I know that this will go on for a long time but I look forward to the day when the pain will not be so intense. I know that life will never be the same as it would have been if the baby had survived, but I hope to one day make some sense of all of this and perhaps even find some meaning for what we are going through."

By addressing the pain, seeking to feel understood and not judged, negotiating painful events, and perhaps discovering some meaning in the loss, grieving parents may find that life will return to normal. Of course this does not mean normal as it was or would have been, but a new normal.

NOTES

1. Schiff, H.S. (1977). The bereaved parent. New York: Crown.
2. Miles, M.S., and Demi, A.S. (1984). Toward the development of a theory of bereavement guilt: Sources of guilt in bereaved parents. Omega 14:299–314.
3. Cook, J.A. (1988). Dad's double binds: Rethinking father's bereavement from a men's studies perspective. Journal of Contemporary Ethnography 17:285–308.
4. Johnson, S. (1984–85). Sexual intimacy and replacement children after the death of a child. Omega 15:109–118.
5. Klass, D. (1986–87). Marriage and divorce among bereaved parents in a self-help group. Omega 17:237–249.
6. Legg, C., and Sherick, I. (1976). The replacement child—a developmental tragedy. Child Psychiatry & Human Development 7:113–126.
7. Poznanski, E.O. (1972). The replacement child: A saga of unresolved parental grief. Journal of Pediatrics 81:1190–1193.
8. Cain, A.C., and Cain, B.S. (1964). On replacing a child. Journal of American Academy of Child Psychiatrists 3:443–456.
9. Klass, D. (1988). Parental grief: Solace and resolution. New York: Springer.
10. Spinetta, J., Swarner, J., and Sheposh, J. (1981). Effective parental coping following the death of a child from cancer. Journal of Pediatric Psychology 6:251–263.

11. Segal, S., Fletcher, M., and Meekison, W.G. (1986). Survey of bereaved parents. Canadian Medical Association Journal 134:38–42.

12. Worden, J.W. (1982). Grief counseling and grief therapy: A handbook for the mental health practitioner. New York: Springer, second edition, 1991.

13. Bernstein, P.P., et al. (1989). Resistance to psychotherapy after a child dies. The effects of the death on parents and siblings. Psychotherapy 26:227–232.

14. Miles, M.A., and Crandall, E.K.B. (1983). The search for meaning and its potential for affecting growth in bereaved parents. Health Values 7:19–21.

15. Alexy, W.D. (1982). Dimensions of psychological counseling that facilitate the growing process of bereaved parents. Journal of Counseling Psychology 29: 498–507.

16. Murphy, S.A., Aroian, K., and Baugher, R.J. (1989). A theory-based preventive intervention program for bereaved parents whose children have died in accidents. Journal of Traumatic Stress 2:319–334.

17. Videka-Sherman, L. (1982). Coping with the death of a child: A study over time. American Journal of Orthopsychiatry 52:688–698.

18. Rubin, S. (1981). A two-track model of bereavement: Theory and application in research. American Journal of Orthopsychiatry 5:101–109.

19. Satir, V. (1988). The new peoplemaking. Mountain View, CA: Science and Behavior Books.

20. Bowlby, J. (1980). Attachment and loss: Loss, sadness, and depression (vol. 3). New York: Basic Books.

21. Videka-Sherman, L., and Lieberman, M. (1985). The effects of self-help and psychotherapy intervention on child loss: The limits of recovery. American Journal of Orthopsychiatry 55:70–82.

8

After a Child Dies:
Helping the Siblings

BETTY DAVIES

A child's death is a critical event for the surviving siblings. This early be-reavement experience may not only affect their emotional development, but also how they cope with similar losses in the future. This chapter describes assumptions that are basic to the concept of sibling bereavement, the re-sponses of children to a sibling's death, some of the factors that influence siblings' grief, and suggests ways in which hospice personnel can help be-reaved siblings.

ASSUMPTIONS BASIC TO SIBLINGS AND GRIEF

Three critical assumptions provide the foundation for understanding sibling grief. First, hospice personnel must fully accept that **children have feelings**. Adults may assume that because children are young, they are unaware and are not affected by a death. Such assumptions mean that, when a child dies, surviving children are often the most neglected family members. They are frequently excluded from the family's mourning by being separated from other family members. Such separation only adds to the children's confusion and to their sense of loneliness and isolation even in the midst of everyday activities.

Second, **children do grieve**. Their grief may be expressed differently from how adults express their grief, but it does exist and it is related to children's comprehension of death at various ages. Children's concepts of death differ from adult views. Each age group has its characteristic ways of understand-ing death, and such guidelines should be reviewed frequently by adults who care for surviving children.

The third assumption is that **sibling relationships are significant**. Most

140

children have at least one sibling with whom they will share a greater part of their life than with any other person. Parents share only 50 to 60% of their children's lifespan, whereas siblings share as much as 80 to 100%. Moreover, siblings spend more time together than any other family subsystem and exert a powerful influence in shaping one another's identity.[1] From the time a new baby enters a family, a special bond develops between the children. Older ones help care for the younger ones, often coaching and teaching them. Children share household tasks, share secrets from their parents and other adults, and defend and protect one another when they are away from the safety of home. When a sibling dies, an emptiness remains that no one else can fill.

IMMEDIATE RESPONSES OF SIBLINGS TO THE CHILD'S DEATH

Context

When a child's death follows a long-term illness, the concept of anticipatory grief leads to the assumption that an "unexpected" death is more difficult for the survivors than an "expected" death. Every child's death, however, is unexpected at the time at which it occurs. After the death, parents and siblings who had accepted the inevitable outcome of the child's illness, have been heard to comment, "But I didn't think he would die until he graduated," "I thought he would wait until I got home from school." Even with preparation time, the actual death is a final surprise. No degree of education or anticipatory grief adequately prepares family members for the reality of death until all bodily functions cease permanently. Anticipatory grief does not replace the grief that follows the actual death.

Shock and Indifference

Children may respond to the news of their sibling's death in ways that adults are totally unprepared for. Although predictable patterns characterize the responses of various age groups, all children are individuals and will respond in their own ways. Therefore, adults must be prepared for each sibling to react to the shock differently. Younger children especially may respond to the news by asking for permission to go and play now. Such reactions are sometimes difficult for parents and other adults if they do not understand that these are normal responses for children. As adults do, children resort to familiar patterns when they hear bad news, or when they are afraid or anxious. To return quickly to the familiarity of playing is a way of gaining some control over what seems like a very scary, uncontrollable situation. Older children attempt to gain some control by seeking refuge in solitude. These children, struggling with independence and with the embarrassment of expressing strong feelings, may respond to the news by running from the room or escaping to a quiet corner or the outdoors. Most important, adults must not judge children's immediate responses as "good" or "bad." Adults must not jump to the conclusion that seemingly indifferent children do not care or did not love the ill child enough.

Guidelines for Telling Siblings About the Death

Depending on the circumstances, hospice caregivers may be the ones to tell the siblings about the death. Several guidelines can be helpful in informing children that their brother or sister has died. First, if it is at all possible, parents are the best ones to tell the siblings. Sometimes, caregivers can be most helpful by supporting the parents in this emotional task. At other times, parents may be too overwhelmed to talk with their children. In these cases, caregivers can give the news to the children, explaining to them that their parents are very saddened, and then reuniting them with their parents as soon as possible: "Your mom and dad are feeling very sad right now. They want to be with you, but they couldn't tell you themselves. Everybody has a different way of reacting to sad news, and that is okay."

When telling children about the death, find a quiet and private place, away from the curiosity of others. Begin with a "warning" of the news that is to come: "I have some sad news for you, Mary," or "You remember that Johnny had difficulty breathing last night?" While conveying the news, sit close to the children, perhaps with a gentle touch, thereby offering reassurance that they are not alone.

Provide the children with a brief but accurate description of what happened. Do not use euphemisms or refer to religious beliefs. Simply say that the child died: "Johnny was sleeping on his bed by the window. Your mother and I had lifted him higher up on the pillows, and we were sitting beside him, when he took one deep breath, and then he died . . . about noon."

Sharing your own feelings with the children is helpful in letting them know that you too are sad, and that it is okay to talk about the shock and sadness: "We all knew that Johnny would not get better, but I still can't believe that he has died. I will miss him very much." Reassure children that their feelings and reactions are okay: "Sometimes we don't know what to do or say, or even how we feel, when we hear this kind of news." Sit quietly with the children and give them time, if they want, to talk or to just absorb the news. If the children want to return to their play, or to be alone, to cry or to scream, respect their wishes, knowing that such responses are "normal."

BEHAVIORAL RESPONSES OF SIBLINGS TO THE CHILD'S DEATH

Short-term Responses

A wide range of behavioral responses tends to occur in siblings after the death of a child. Since children often work out their feelings through their behaviors, and since behavior represents a relatively easy way of assessing children's responses to critical events, it is logical that the focus of much research in this area has been on behavior.

Following the death, siblings may demonstrate a range of psychophysiological behaviors, most of which are similar to the grief responses of adults. Children complain of frequent headaches, tummy aches, or other aches and pains. They often have sleeping difficulties; they may resist going to bed or may fear the dark. This is particularly true for siblings who shared a room with their sibling. Other children wake up frequently, telling of nightmares or bad dreams. Some children have disturbances in appetite, either not wanting to eat, or eating too much. Children may show increased anxiety, especially about getting involved in new activities, especially for children whose primary companion was their sibling. When siblings themselves are sick, they are often unusually anxious about being alone and about having to go to the hospital.

Other children may act out and become aggressive, irritable, and argumentative, putting an extra strain on interactions with their parents. Many are sad, lonely, and withdrawn. Most children experience some decreased ability to concentrate and, as a result, their school work may suffer.

The developmental differences that characterize children's understanding of death also characterize children's responses to grief. In addition to the behavioral responses described above, children in each age group may respond in ways outlined in Table 8.1.

A standardized behavioral checklist was used to assess the responses of children whose sibling had died within the past three years.[2] Summary scores indicated that the bereaved siblings had overall higher total behavior problem scores, particularly for internalizing behaviors, than the standardized norms. Moreover, the social competency scores were lower than what the standardized norms predicted, and these scores decreased over time. These findings suggest that if a sibling demonstrates a pattern of behavior which includes persistent sadness and withdrawal, decreased involvement

Table 8.1   Behavioral Responses According to Age

Ages 2–5

- Children may be clinging, fearful to be away from parents or to try new activities.
- May repeat questions which reflect that they are trying to understand what "dead" means: When will Johnny be back? Will God make Johnny better and send him back? Can we go to see Johnny now?
- Due to their magical thinking, children may fear that something they did caused the death. Similarly, they imagine that their behavior, such as being very good, might bring Johnny back.
- Children's play may express thoughts and feelings and center around the reenactment of events such as the funeral.

Ages 6–9

- Due to the common preoccupation with the "scary" aspects of death, children may be fearful of monsters in their room, of ghosts, and of the bogeyman coming to get them (or their parents).
- When death is discussed and not knowing how to respond, they may act silly or laugh or suddenly become very quiet. This applies particularly to the surviving children's playmates, whose behavior then adds to the sadness of the grieving children.
- Fearful that their parents may also die, children may show increased interest in staying at home or in their parents' health and well being.
- Children's play may involve violence, such as having cars crash and burn.

Ages 9–12

- Self-conscious about expressing their feelings and about their behavior, preteens do not want to seem different from their peers.
- They may ask for guidance about how to act and what to say.
- Children may be judgmental about their own behavior and that of others, getting upset with "gross" displays of emotion.

Ages 12–15

- Feeling that their emotions are in turmoil, they may show extremes of behavior, hysterically crying one minute followed by embarrassed laughter the next.
- Embarrassed to show their emotions in front of their friends, they may isolate themselves or go to great lengths to give the impression that "everything is fine."

in activities and hobbies, persistent acting out, diminished self-esteem, and a loss of interest and achievement in school, the child should be given individual attention through referral to the school counselor or to a specialist in children's grief.

Long-term Responses

Persistent Effects

Most studies of sibling bereavement and, in fact, most bereavement studies focus on the months immediately after the death, or up to one or two years following the death. Consequently, the long-term effects of sibling bereavement are relatively unknown. Awareness of the long-term effects emphasizes that siblings, in addition to parents, must receive the careful attention of hospice personnel.

In follow-up studies of siblings who experienced the death of a brother or sister in childhood, siblings reported ongoing effects.[3] Several siblings continued to dream about the deceased brother or sister. They did not find the dreams disturbing but rather comforting in that they provided feelings of closeness to the deceased sibling. Feelings of loneliness and sadness persisted. Many siblings continued to think about their siblings frequently, sometimes as often as once a day. Such thoughts were triggered by internal and external reminders. Internal reminders stemmed from the siblings' thoughts about events in their own lives, such as reaching the age at which their sibling had died: "You can't just sit back and say, 'Well, I don't have to worry about dying until I'm eighty' . . . because he was only seventeen, like I am now. That does bother me. I think back and I'm not at all prepared for death like he was at this age." External reminders included seeing photographs, letters, or other people who reminded them of their sibling, hearing conversations about the sibling, or songs that rekindled memories: "I would be driving down the road in my car and they played 'Dust in the Wind' . . . 'all we are is dust in the wind'. I would have to pull over because I would be crying so much." Having children of their own also stimulated poignant memories of the deceased sibling.

Up to ten, twenty, or thirty years after the death, siblings reported that the death still had an ongoing impact on their lives, often a constant reminder about the value of life. It is critical to note that the long-term effects of sibling bereavement are not necessarily pathological, even though periods of intense sadness may recur years later. Some individuals, particularly those who had experienced sibling death during adolescence, felt that the long-term effects had been detrimental to their development.[4] For these individuals, their newly found maturity at a young age was accompanied by a seriousness about life that left little room for the normal developmental antics of childhood and adolescence. The natural tendency to withdraw into oneself that accompanies grief was compounded by a sense of intolerance for peer activities, and the withdrawal was enhanced. As a result, siblings were often lonely. Moreover, their withdrawal had removed them from situations on learning how to socialize with their peers. They had "missed out" on learning how to foster social relationships during a critical period of development. As adults, their loneliness persisted.

Growth-promoting Effects

The enduring effects of losing a sibling are not only potentially negative; although painful, the experience may provide children with the impetus for psychological growth. In one study, siblings scored higher on a measure of self-concept (the Piers-Harris Self-Concept Scale for Children) than the normative group of children.[5] Correlations between the Piers-Harris scores and length of illness, time elapsed since death, and age and sex of the siblings were not significant.

Looking back, many siblings perceived positive outcomes of the experience that may have contributed to their higher self-concepts. Siblings felt comfortable with death and were able to help, instead of avoid, other individuals who were undergoing a death-related event. Siblings reported that their experience facilitated the development of a sensitive outlook on life, and siblings generally felt good about what they had learned. These findings offer some reassurance that the death of a sibling does not have only long-term negative effects for the surviving children. As occurs with any traumatic experience, there is also potential for growth as a possible outcome.

FACTORS THAT INFLUENCE CHILDREN'S GRIEF

Not all children react in the same way to the death of a sibling. It is, therefore, helpful for hospice personnel to know what factors should be considered in assessing children's reaction to the death of their brother or sister. Location of death is frequently described as pertinent to bereavement outcome in children following the long-term illness of a sibling. In addition, however, there are other factors that come into play, regardless of the place of death, and help to mediate the effects of the death on siblings.

Place of Death

If given a choice, most ill children prefer to be with their parents, their families and friends, and among familiar belongings at home. When children are dying, their preference for home care is even stronger. Some families may not choose home care, but for those who do, home care has been remarkably effective from the perspective of the siblings following the child's death.

Studies examining the differential adjustment of siblings have shown that a child's death at home has benefits over death in a hospital. The behavior reactions of children three to twenty-nine months following a sibling's death at home were within normal limits on a standardized checklist, whereas those children whose sibling had died in a hospital had higher scores of fear and neurotic behavior.[6] Moreover, one year after the death, siblings described a significantly different experience depending on the place of death. Those whose siblings had died in a hospital generally described themselves as having been inadequately prepared for the death, isolated from the dying child and their parents, unable to use their parents for support information, unclear as to the circumstances of the death, and useless in terms of their own involvement.[7] In contrast, siblings of children who died at home were prepared for the impending death, received consistent information and support from their parents, were involved in most activities concerning the dying child, were present for the death, and viewed their own involvement as the most important aspect of the experience.

Shared Life Space

Bereavement outcome seems to have a lot to do with how much of each other's life space the deceased person and the survivor have occupied.[8] This is particularly true for siblings who were emotionally close to their brother or sister.[9] Siblings who had such predeath relationships tended to demonstrate more internalizing behavior (sadness, withdrawal) after the child's death. Emotional closeness between siblings exerted a stronger influence on bereavement outcome than closeness in age, length of illness, or number of surviving children in the family. For example, the relationship between 15-year-old Cameron and his 4-year-old sister, Jennifer, was the "closest" sibling relationship in their family of four children. Because of their age and sex differences, Cameron and Jennifer shared few belongings and spent relatively little time together. Cameron doted on his little sister, however, and in the words of his mother, he "opened up more to his little sister than to anyone." They shared a very special closeness. After Jennifer died, Cameron scored at the 87th percentile on the "Uncommunicative or Social Withdrawal" subscale of the behavior checklist. Hospice personnel therefore need to be particularly sensitive to those children who shared a close relationship with their brother or sister.

Family Environment

The family is critical in creating an environment that may affect children's responses to the death of a sibling. The family provides for its members the necessary relationships, in terms of both quality and intensity, through which normal growth and development occur.

In one study, findings indicated that families, who were more cohesive and active in social and recreational activities and who put a greater emphasis on religious aspects, had children who demonstrated fewer behavioral problems up to three years after the death of a sibling from cancer.[2] One family, for example, had relocated to a different region of the country four years previously, and still had not established any new friendships. They did not participate in any activities outside of their home. When their son died, the family used the Yellow Pages to identify a minister to conduct the funeral. Neither the parents nor the surviving 16-year-old daughter could recall any of the son's friends attending the service. Of all participating families, this family had the lowest score on two subscales of the Family Environment Scale: the Active/Recreational Orientation and the Intellectual/Cultural Orientation subscales. Moreover, the surviving child had dropped out of school and was presenting numerous behavioral problems as evidenced by her high score on the behavioral checklist. In contrast was the family with the highest scores on the same two subscales. When their son died, several relatives came immediately from far distances to be with the family. Numerous friends from the local church, the community, and the children's school had attended the funeral. The surviving child in this family had very few behavioral problems and he was doing extremely well in school and in his social relationships.

These findings indicated that the social support gained by having a family emphasis on social, recreational, and religious activities seemed to serve a protective function for children who experienced the death of a sibling. In their attempt to help bereaved siblings, clinicians therefore need to pay attention to the family unit, showing sensitivity to the amount of social support that families have. In those families with little support, hospice workers often become a vital source of support and can facilitate family involvement in community-based support groups before and after the death of their child.

Sibling Perceptions of Status in the Family

How children perceive their own value, in relation to the child who died, is a critical variable in sibling bereavement. Earlier, reference was made to a study of self-concept in bereaved siblings.[5] Within the total group, some children had higher self-concept scores than others. Content analysis of the sibling interviews indicated a possible explanation for this difference: the feeling of "I'm not enough" in children with the lower self-concept scores. This feeling was clearly evident in the children with the lower scores and was clearly absent in the children with the higher scores.

Children felt this way when they perceived that they compared favorably with the child who died. And, of most interest, was that this feeling existed before the child died or had even become ill. Seven-year-old Mary, for example, "could never figure out why Grandma liked Marc [the deceased child] more than she liked me." Grandma had always shown preferential treatment to Marc, bringing him gifts even on Mary's birthday. Mary felt as though she should have been the one to die, since Marc had so much more to offer the family. In some families, the parents' preference for one child over the other validated the children's perceptions of not "being enough." For some children, their sense of less worth was enhanced when they sensed that they were in some way responsible for the death, such as by bringing home the common cold or chicken pox.

In contrast, the parents of children with high self-concept scores gave no indication that the surviving children were not as good as the deceased child, nor did they even hint at blaming the surviving children in any way. These parents talked proudly about each of their children, not for their accomplishments but just for being who they were. They also were explicit about telling their children how much they were loved. Each child was considered special.

Surviving children also felt as though they were "not enough" when they felt displaced by other children. When surviving children perceived that the newcomers were substitutes for the deceased child, then they thought, "If I were enough, Mom and Dad wouldn't need another baby."

The feeling of "I'm not enough" was manifested in two patterns of sibling behavior: overachieving and parental caregiving. Overachieving was evident in schoolwork or in children taking on extra jobs and responsibilities. Many children were described as more caring, thoughtful, and mature as a result of their experience with death. However, the object of their caregiving differed between the child with high and low self-concepts. The children with the highest scores directed their caregiving in age-appropriate ways to younger siblings or to peers. Those children with the lowest scores took on adult responsibilities by becoming the caregivers of their parents.

Hospice personnel therefore must be sensitive to family interactions and support attempts at ways of improving parent-child relationships during and after the death of a child. While recognizing that parents feel exhausted and overburdened while their child is ill, and experience intense grief when the child dies, hospice personnel can be instrumental in devising ways of helping parents see each of their children as special, and to role model and reinforce expressions of caring for all children.

GUIDELINES FOR HELPING SIBLINGS AND FAMILIES

Two critical assumptions provide the foundation for helping bereaved siblings. First, hospice workers must recognize the impact of a child's death on the siblings so that these children in fact receive the necessary attention. Second, hospice personnel must remember that parents are the best persons to help their children. This is not to say that direct contact by hospice caregivers with the siblings is not important; only that the parents are the ones who set the tone in the family for dealing with the death and for letting the siblings know that they too are special.

Supporting the Parents

The way in which children work through their grief depends a lot on how their parents and other adults handle themselves and reach out to them. The better the parents are able to cope, the better it will be for the children. The most valuable assistance for the children therefore may be to support the parents in their grief and to offer them assistance in how to help their children (Table 8.2). Also, by maintaining some sense of stability within the family, parents will make things a lot easier for their children. This is not an easy thing for parents to do, and they may need to be encouraged to go for help or to accept the help that is being offered.

Sometimes parents are so overwhelmed with their own grief, and with other stressful life events, that they cannot deal with their children's grief. In such cases, parents need to be reassured that this too is an acceptable response, and that they will be able to help their children when they themselves feel better. Meanwhile, parents can suggest the names of other adults, familiar to the children, who are willing to be available to give special attention to the children. An adult should be identified for each child in the

Table 8.2   Guidelines for Helping Grieving Siblings

- Spend time with children, explaining again and again what happened and answering their questions.
- Share your own memories and feelings with children.
- Use physical touch as a way of reassuring and comforting children.
- Tell children how much the deceased child loved them.
- Reassure children that it is not likely that anyone else (particularly the parents) will also die within the near future.
- Encourage children to express their own feelings and thoughts in their own ways.
- Continue to allow the child to have responsibilities around the house as a way of "normalizing" life.
- Give simple directions or utilize reminder lists for things that need to be done (children, as well as adults, have a hard time remembering while they are grieving).
- Encourage children's involvement with their friends and peers.
- Recognize that there are no magic words. Avoid saying "I know how you feel."
- Avoid comparisons between the surviving children and the deceased sibling.
- Let children know that feeling sad, angry, or scared is okay for adults and for children, and that crying is okay (even for boys).
- Allow laughter and fun times, which do occur even in the midst of great sadness.

---

family. These adults should be asked to take on this special role, with an explanation of how important the role is, and the children should be included in the decision.

Involving the Children

Basic to involving children in the grief process is the belief that children are persons with rights to know what is happening, to participate in family events, both joyful and sad, and to express grief in their own ways. Children should be given opportunities to help in planning and participating in the funeral or other family rituals, to the degree that they wish. In order to allow children to make the best choices, however, they need to be given explanations about what will happen and what to expect. They also must know that their input and assistance is needed and desired. For example, younger children can answer the doorbell or pass cookies when people visit. Older children can answer the phone. Teenagers can pick up relatives at the airport or go on errands.

As time goes on, the children need also to participate in decisions about what to do with the deceased child's belongings. In families where the individual memories associated with various belongings were shared openly among family members, the children demonstrated fewer behavioral problems following their sibling's death.[10] Discussions about how to handle anniversary dates, the child's birthday, and other special occasions need to be ongoing between parents and children.

Expressing Emotions

Helping children deal with the sadness and anger they feel after a death is one of the most difficult challenges adults face in helping grieving siblings. Children may feel waves of sadness following their sibling's death, made worse by feelings of loneliness. Even though children may understand that their sibling's illness is not curable, after the death, they may feel angry at their parents, the doctors and nurses, or God for not being able to at least postpone the death. Their anger may be fueled by the disruption in their lives following the death or by the lack of control over their own emotions. Since anger is often the result of guilt, it is also important to reassure children that nothing they said, did, or imagined was responsible for causing the child to die. Ensure that children are aware of the events that occurred at the time of death. Sometimes, the guilt stems from not having said good-bye. When this is the case, children can be encouraged to express the good-bye they would have said by writing a letter, drawing a picture, or verbalizing to a photo of the deceased child.

One way to deal with these emotions is to encourage children to express how sad or angry they are and to find an outlet for these feelings. An effective strategy is for adults to share their own feelings with their children: "I feel so mad sometimes because Johnny died. We all tried so hard to make him better, and he didn't want to die. I sometimes wonder why he couldn't have got better, or at least, have lived for a little while longer. It's normal to feel this way. . . . I know we can't stop the feelings, but we can do something about them. I've been scrubbing the floor (hitting golf balls, digging in the garden) a lot lately, and that does help me get rid of these mad feelings." Being honest with children in this way not only normalizes the children's feelings, it also lets them know that their parents share similar feelings, and that there are constructive ways to handle the feelings.

CONCLUSION

The death of a child is a traumatic event for siblings. The intensity of the immediate impact results in a range of behavioral responses which do seem to diminish over time. The experience is mediated by a variety of factors, some of which have been described. In helping siblings, what hospice personnel must remember most is that the goal of intervention is not for siblings to get over their grief, but rather to acknowledge it and to learn to integrate it into their lives, for it is a memory that they carry with them forever.

NOTES

1. Bank, S. & Kahn, M.D. (1982). The sibling bond. New York: Basic Books.

2. Davies, B. (1988). The family environment in bereaved families and its relationship to surviving sibling behaviour. Children's Health Care 17:22–30.

3. Davies, B. (1990). Long-term follow-up of bereaved siblings. In Morgan, J. (Ed.), The dying and bereaved teenager. Philadelphia: Charles Press.

4. Davies, B. (1991). Long-term outcomes of adolescent sibling bereavement. Journal of Adolescent Research 6:83–96.

5. Martinson, I.M., Davies, E.B., & McClowry, S.G. (1987). The long-term effects of sibling death on self-concept. Journal of Pediatric Nursing 2:227–235.

6. Mulhern, R.K., Lauer, M.E., & Hoffman, R.G. (1983). Death of a child at home or in the hospital: Subsequent psychological adjustment of the family. Pediatrics 71:743–747.

7. Lauer, M.E., Mulhern, R.K., Bohne, J.B., & Camitta, B.M. (1985). Children's perceptions of their siblings' death at home or hospital. The precursors of differential adjustment. Cancer Nursing 6:21–27.

8. Parkes, C.M. (1972). Bereavement: Studies of grief in adult life. New York: International Universities Press.

9. Davies, B. (1988). Shared life space and sibling bereavement responses. Cancer Nursing 11:339–347.

10. Davies, B. (1987). Family responses to the death of a child: The meaning of memories. Journal of Palliative Care 3:9–15.

9

Lessons in Grief:
A Practical Look at School Programs

ELLEN GORTLER

A first-grader dies six weeks into the school year after a one-and-a-half year battle with leukemia. An 8-year-old is hit by a car. The space shuttle *Challenger* explodes, killing a schoolteacher as her class watches on television. A high school junior commits suicide. *Operation Desert Storm* calls to arms nearly half a million service men and women, leaving their families and neighbors to ponder the unthinkable. High school students rank among those at highest risk for HIV infection.

Schoolchildren and faculty regularly face death and other traumatic losses in our increasingly complex society. Real violence erupts on the streets, in stark contrast to television's fantasies. Drug abuse plagues our schools. Students grapple with their parents' divorces when they should be tackling algebra. Across America, situations like these are forcing school faculties and administrators to consider grief programs that help children to understand and cope with feelings of loss.

PERSPECTIVE

Grief is nothing new for children. To the contrary, less than a hundred years ago children experienced life, in all of its splendor and devastation, side by side with adults. Before the modernization of health care, before life-prolonging technology for the very old and oh-so-young, and before death itself seemed a medical or human failure, rather than the natural end to life that it is, birth and death, aging and sickness occurred at home—right there—in front of the children. Children used to experience life in a way that legitimized death and grief. Now they are ill-prepared, protected by modern technology and a culture that says children should be shielded from selected aspects of life's realities.

154

Pioneers in death education began highlighting these observations in the early 1960s to expose ours as a death-denying society. In the 1977 premiere issue of *Death Education*, Herman Feifel traces modern America's ambivalence to death.[1] From biblical times until as recently as our grandparents' memories, society's beliefs about death were steeped in religion; death was but a door to a better existence. Today our modern secularism stresses youth, convenience, immortality through personal achievement, and medical miracles. We think we have beaten the Grim Reaper. There is no room for him in our thinking. The professionalization of many family matters— among them illness, dying, and death—has also worked to push him even further out of sight.

Although the death-education concept emerged as an academic pursuit, reaching its heyday in the 1970s on college campuses and in some high-school classrooms, it was not until the mid-1980s that programs for primary and secondary schools became widely available. Yet despite broad growth in the field, a 1990 report of the Association for Death Education and Counseling showed that only 17% of public schools surveyed offered a grief education or support program, and only 11% taught general death education courses.[2] The number of suicide intervention and prevention programs came in slightly higher at 25%.

These findings are strikingly similar to those of the decade before, a fact that reseachers Hannerlore Wass and colleagues reported to be particularly disappointing given the increasing needs of today's children, the depth of knowledge now available to school staffs, and the proven benefits to children when schools actively participate in death and grief support programs.[2] The authors point to a lingering "death avoidance" in our society and the need for more academic preservice or professional in-service training to better prepare school faculty for addressing this reality of life.

SKELETONS OF CONTROVERSY

Of course most of our death avoidance is a natural reaction to life's ultimate threat. However, some of the phenomena experienced in today's schools may stem in part from memories of controversy and criticism surrounding public school death education programs during the last fifteen years. Controversy has centered on two issues, both, ironically, a result of the subject's growing acceptance. An additional irony is that a good many of the critics have been long-time proponents of death education—but only of programs provided by appropriately trained professionals. Many anticipated the pitfalls associated with allowing death education to become too available and were first in line to criticize those pitfalls that did emerge.[3-9]

Concern one: *In promoting acceptance of death and coping techniques, an overzealous program or facilitator can, in fact, aid in the denial process with sometimes-dangerous results.*[3,4,7,9] Rare, tragic cases have been reported in which some high school students were so enchanted with death that they tried, sometimes successfully, to take their own lives.[3,9] These courses tended to concentrate on now-avoided, emotionally charged aspects of dying that encouraged students to imagine different types of death and even try coffins on for size. Regarding another aspect of this issue, some critics have warned that by its very nature—pigeon-holing death and grief processes into manageable stages and snappy terminology—death education can entrap students into an academic or cognitive denial. Thus, if a program is too successful in making death acceptable, it could rob grief of its emotional depth and life-changing impact. Some critics suggest that this can cause a numbing effect that leaves students prone to risk-taking behaviors.[4]

Concern two: *Widely available, preprepared programs give the impression that anyone can effectively teach death, grief, and loss.*[3-7] Death education as an academic pursuit has reached a certain maturity. The dangerous outcome of such maturity, the academics forewarned, can be likened to the mass marketing of hamburgers, causing them to lose their original flavor.[5] There has also been a prevailing fear among this group, stated and implied, that the field will fall into the hands of novices who do not have the education, training, or emotional fortitude to adequately teach such complex and important subject matter to our children.[6]

If ours is a death-denying culture, then the prospect of educating our children in the particulars of the subject must be, by definition, controversial. Should we avoid presenting death and grief issues to children altogether because some may misunderstand or find it too morbid? Should access to current knowledge through prepackaged educational and guidance programs be curtailed in the interest of academic purity?

GRIEF, LOSS, HOSPICE, AND SCHOOLS

Perhaps in answer to prevailing concerns, today's most popular programs for children and those who teach them focus on the psychologic components of grief and loss. Physiologic aspects of death are addressed as necessary for an understanding of death as a permanent, lifeless condition. However, one is challenged to find even the term *death education* among modern "grief and loss" programs for schoolchildren. Another advantage to generalized grief programs is that they address other aspects of loss that are so pervasive in our children's world, among them divorce, serious illness, injury, and even moving. In addition, there is an increased emphasis on providing training and ongoing support to ensure faculty preparedness for effective presentation of such complex subject matter and the issues that may subsequently arise.

Hospice has had significant impact on school programs throughout the country. Often a community's only resource on grief, loss, and children, hospice programs have been in the unique position to offer this expertise for the school setting. Many hospice programs begin in this role as a natural extension of a patient's care. At other times the hospice staff is approached by a school administrator or faculty member at a time of crisis. However, with more and more frequency, hospice is taking an active role in assessing the needs of the community as a whole and of local schools in particular. School administrators and faculty are also becoming more aware of their role in helping children cope in an increasingly complex world. Despite claims of already overgenerous curricula and inadequate budgets, many school faculties are recognizing the need to incorporate grief and loss concepts into guidance or health programs.

Although no two programs are exactly alike, they incorporate many of the same components, tapping the growing body of knowledge on children and grief. Most fall within the range of two categories: direct classroom or guidance curricula for children, and facilitative programs for school faculties. Many incorporate both curricula and provider training. The most comprehensive programs provide on-site instruction, facilitators' guides and session plans, a choice of student activities, and necessary collateral materials. The simplest programs take the form of practical facilitators' guides, children's activity books, or audio-visual material for use alone or in conjunction with programs already in place.

PROGRAM COMPONENTS

Early on, all programs define *loss* and validate the range of emotion that comes with it. Depending on the program's focus, sources of loss are identified with emphasis on death of a loved one, separation caused by divorce, serious injury or illness, and trauma associated with moving. At this time, a session may also address physical aspects of death or illness. Programs often employ an ice-breaking activity to help participants explore their own experiences, including fear and anxiety. The purpose of this type of activity is threefold. First, it imparts an understanding of the loss concept. Second, it encourages discussion of taboo subject matter, often for the first time in the participant's life. Finally, it promotes the listening skills necessary to help a grieving individual. Activities of this kind are particularly important for potential program facilitators, since a teacher's effectiveness in helping children cope with loss can be largely dependent on his or her own ability to come to grips with it.[10–12]

Most programs define and distinguish among grief, mourning, and bereavement. *Grief* is the individual, psychologic, and somatic reaction to the death of a loved one or another significant loss. *Mourning* is the sharing of grief in a supportive environment, incorporating beliefs, traditions, and ceremonies. *Bereavement* is the state of separation caused by a loss. The grief process, often called "grief work," is usually defined. Although controversial because it locks grief into a linear model, most grief programs' definitions are based at least in part on Elisabeth Kübler-Ross' five stages of death, dying, and the grief experience: denial and isolation, anger, bargaining, depression and withdrawal, and acceptance.[13]

Incorporated into basic definitions are theories of cognitive development that affect a student's ability to understand and cope with loss depending on age. For instance, it is widely recognized that children's understanding of death occurs in four stages.[14,15] The child who experiences a significant loss must then cognitively revisit and explore that loss experience during each subsequent stage in development.

In infancy, no conceptualization of death is believed to occur, although even the youngest children feel the effects of separation. Children first begin to understand death between the ages of 3 and 5, but to the young child, death is a reversible condition much like sleep. Preschoolers often partake in magical thinking and believe in their ability to make things happen just by wishing them so. This can result in unwarranted feelings of guilt if a loss should occur after a child has wished someone would "go away."

Later in childhood—from ages 6 to 9—a child begins to understand that death is permanent, but tends to personify death as an angel or ghost. Because of the child's increasing sense of personal power at this age, most children do not believe that death could ever happen to them. There is also a normal, although seemingly morbid, interest in the physiologic aspects of death for this age group.

Between the ages of 10 and 12, most children are capable of understanding death as irreversible, universal, and inevitable. During adolescence children realize that death can happen to anyone, regardless of age, and adapt their own philosophies and belief systems concerning their vulnerability. At this anxious stage, children joke about death, tell ghost stories, and may challenge their own mortality by taking excessive risks.

The impact of any children's grief program is realized by its ability to foster a supportive environment in which participants can explore grief experiences within the context of these developmental stages. Some programs use art, literature, music, and role-playing to demonstrate human commonalities and cultural differences in grief behavior and customs. In addition, programs identify and emphasize the value of support networks that help children cope with loss. These include family, friends, teachers, and professional community resources. An objective of most programs is to take theory one step further by encouraging positive behaviors and teaching coping skills.

Among the *do's* and *don'ts* recommended for teachers discussing death with children:[16,17]

- Let children express their feelings. Do not tell them to "be brave."
- Use simple and direct language about death, remembering the children's developmental level. For example: "Karen has died. She can never come back to school, but we will always remember her."
- Avoid complicated explanations. Begin with information that is the least emotional.
- Reassure children that they are not responsible for a death. Dispel any magical thoughts that could lead children to this conclusion.
- When serious illness is the cause of death, remind children that this is quite different from common colds or minor illnesses.
- Present information in a nonmoralistic fashion. It is best for teachers to discuss religious topics in the context of what different groups of people do. Recommend that children discuss beliefs with their families.
- Be sensitive to emotional or negative reactions to the information presented. Sometimes these can be therapeutic. Use professional judgment in referring a child for further counseling.
- Do not use euphemisms. Associating death with sleep or a long trip can make children fearful of everyday occurrences.
- Admit that some things cannot be understood about death. Nobody has all of the answers.

THE SERIOUSLY ILL CHILD

Several specialized programs address issues pertaining to seriously ill children. As survival rates for childhood cancers have increased markedly in the last thirty years, much has been written about the reentry of the seriously ill child into the school setting and the need for schools to effectively and compassionately assimilate these children back into the classroom. The growing incidence and risks of HIV and AIDS infection among the school-age population further complicates the responsibilities of school systems to meet the needs of the ill child and classmates.

Academic and social success at school often comprises the very essence of the seriously ill child's self-esteem and sense of future. However, school management of these children can be fraught with barriers as a result of protective reactions of the child, family, teachers, and schoolmates and their parents.[18] For the child, these reactions are based on his or her perceived inability to perform in school or be accepted into the school setting. For the family, they are a natural urge to shield their child from further stress or exposure to common illnesses that would compromise his or her condition. For educators, it is the human reaction to childhood illness and mortality that is intensified by their own questions of preparedness to address the issues. For schoolmates, it is an age-appropriate grief reaction magnified by their own anxiety and curiosity. And, finally, parents of the student body add to these reactions the desire to protect their own children from such unhappy circumstances or possible illness. Key to a school's fulfillment of so vital a role is careful preparation, openness to understanding, and anticipation of needs for all affected by the child's illness.

It is generally recommended that school professionals first meet with the child's parents, health-care professionals, and the child so that the child's condition can be fully understood. Teachers and other school staff can then anticipate the child's physical, social, and academic needs and promptly meet them.[19,20,21] The needs and wishes of the child and the family, including siblings, also demand active consideration.

The seriously ill child and the family are already experiencing grief reactions to the child's condition; the assault of catastrophic illness and frequent hospitalizations on all aspects of family life are well documented. In addition to such normal grief feelings as shock, denial, and anger, parents often feel guilt, loss of control, and isolation. They may want to further isolate themselves and their child from any additional stress or harm. Frequent contact with parents throughout a child's illness is imperative to maintaining an ongoing assessment of the family's needs and desires pertaining to their child's school experience. Should the child die, it is especially important to maintain this contact as a show of personal, professional, and community support.[18]

In the same way that grief experiences are tied to a child's stages of cognitive development, so is the seriously ill child's own reactions and ability to understand his or her illness and the changes it inflicts.[22] For example, a preschooler might incorrectly associate the illness with bad behavior, and therefore perceive hospitalization as abandonment and treatment as punishment. The school-age child has a growing understanding of cause and effect and so would be more likely to cooperate with all aspects of care as a means of achieving a goal. However, it should be especially noted among educators that since school is the major accomplishment of children ages 6 to 12, a child's self-esteem at this age is most closely dependent on teacher reactions and a sense of belonging at school.[20] Adolescents and teenagers come with their own set of developmental challenges, regardless of health. The importance of peers, communication, appearance, and independence cannot be overlooked when an adolescent is ill. Issues of body image, mobility, peer acceptance, and privacy are generally of more concern to this age group than the physical discomforts of illness.

Once the needs and wishes of the child and the family are known, the school staff can then extend their focus of preparation to themselves, and the student body and their parents. Since the comfort and ability of the school staff to handle grief-intense situations has been linked to their ultimate success, many recommend special meetings and workshops to familiarize educators with the child's condition, as well as more generalized grief issues. Parents of schoolmates also have the right and need to know when their children are faced with circumstances of such emotional impact. Letters, meetings, and workshops are all recommended ways in which to inform and communicate with the parents of the student body.

Finally, feelings of grief, fear, and anxiety experienced by the student body can be explored by means of the types of guidance and instructional programs that are the subject of this chapter. Participation in such programs has been demonstrated to foster greater understanding between the ill child and schoolmates, and therefore heighten acceptance of the seriously ill child. As with other aspects of planning under such circumstances, particular sensitivity to the wishes of the child and the family should be observed in how a program is implemented and the appropriateness of the program content as it relates to the child's condition.

NECESSITY BREEDS PRACTICALITY: THREE CASES

Whether by means of formal study or informal, even unexpected, response to existing bereavement services, community hospice programs are finding there is a need for grief and loss programs in the schools. *But how does a hospice program assess and fill grief education needs at school?* That depends.

The Case for Spontaneity

In 1990 at Hospice of the Chesapeake, a program of hospice for children and adults in Millersville, Maryland, Bereavement Director Betty Asplund wanted to preview a video on children and grief before she committed program resources to purchase it. She notified a few public school guidance counselors, asking them to pass the word, then set up two viewings with the hope that enough people would attend to give her some feedback. Ms.

Asplund plugged in a coffee pot and hoped for the best. Within minutes their small facility was jammed with interested counselors from all over the county; more than sixty people attended the previews.

Admittedly taken aback, but alerted to a need for resources in the school system, Ms. Asplund and the hospice staff offered a conference, *Children in Grief*, later that year to educators as well as their regular audience of caretakers and clergy. Once again, response confirmed need—approximately 45% of conference attendees were school guidance counselors. As a result, Hospice of the Chesapeake offers support on an as-needed basis to Anne Arundel County Public Schools by way of crisis intervention, support groups, special programs, resource provision, and facilitator support.

By culling resources from a variety of available materials, hospice staff is able to meet the many needs of children throughout their community. Among their often-used resources is the *Bereavement Support Group Program for Children*, a facilitator's guide and participant workbook developed by Beth Haasl and Jean Marnocha at the Bellin Hospice Program in Green Bay, Wisconsin. Hospice of the Chesapeake staff finds this program effective in both support group and school guidance settings.

Also in response to community need, Ms. Asplund has created *Camp Nabe*, a weekend retreat for bereaved children in Anne Arundel County. Using a variety of resources and a staff of professionals and trained volunteers, the camp program acquaints children with grief in general, focusing on anger and guilt—two of the most prevalent grief feelings that children experience. *Camp Nabe*'s program emphasizes that children do not have to be alone in their grief and helps them to identify and enlarge their support system. A facilitator's manual for Camp Nabe is available.

The Case for Careful Planning

Of course, community-needs assessment can benefit from a planned approach. In 1987, Hospice at Greensboro, a program of hospice care for all ages in North Carolina, convened a *Community Task Force on Children and Grief* in an effort to heighten community awareness concerning the needs of grieving children. In addition, hospice staff hoped to gain input and assistance from community professionals and organizations, including the school board, in identifying and funding the best program model for helping children in their community understand and cope with loss. The Task Force looked at programs from three models: support group, support group center, and a school-centered approach. They ultimately chose the school-centered program, *Children and Grief: Living with Loss*. This comprehensive facilitator training and intervention program was developed by Jessica Gurvit while she was the executive director for Hospice of Northeast Jacksonville, Florida.

After securing a grant from the Junior League of Greensboro, hospice staff hired a program facilitator to oversee aspects including training offered to school personnel. Greensboro City schools were the first to participate in 1989. Since 1990, the program has expanded to include the entire Guilford County school system, including High Point City schools.

Adapting the program package to meet their community's needs was another goal of Hospice at Greensboro. As a component of *Living with Loss*, in 1989 the hospice staff and volunteers developed a puppet show based on *Aarvy Aardvark Finds Hope*, Donna O'Toole's book about loss for children. Used as an identification and teaching tool, the popular production is taken on the road annually to third-grade students throughout Guilford County. In 1990 the puppet show received the National Hospice Award for Excellence.

Hospice at Greensboro has since expanded its community outreach with *Kaleidoscope*, a comprehensive pediatric hospice program that serves as an umbrella for all of its children's services. *Kaleidoscope* was established in 1979 by Cynthia Simpson-Byrne at Hospice of Charleston, South Carolina. In addition to *Living with Loss*, the *Aarvy Aardvark Finds Hope* puppet show, and home pediatric hospice care, Greensboro's *Kaleidoscope* program offers *Reaching for Rainbows*, a camp for children who have experienced loss through death, and support groups and counseling for grieving children, youth, and their families.

The Case for Innovation

In Indiana, Hospice of Bloomington Director Carol Ebeling has taken her expertise on children and grief into the schools via video cassette. As hospice director she had worked extensively with schools, as well as with children, families, and the community in times of crisis. Her *Griefbusters of Bloomington* after-school bereavement support group had earned her the community's 1990 *Quality of Life* award, but the many calls she received from local schools illustrated the need to further address school staff preparedness in the event that "grief comes to school."

Available since 1991, *When Grief Comes to School* is a videotaped series of interviews with local school faculty, a bereaved mother, and a bereaved son, interwoven with topical presentations by Ms. Ebeling. The 69-minute program is divided into four sessions for presentation to school faculty and includes a leader's manual with materials for worksheets and transparencies. Practical information presented about the nature of grief and bereavement stresses the needs of those who have experienced death during the immediate grief period and its aftermath. It also gives simple suggestions that schools can use in order to develop a crisis plan.

Ms. Ebeling often provides follow-up consultation and workshops to support schools in applying and expanding on concepts presented in the video. She also encourages school staffs to consult hospice programs in their area.

After its first year, nearly 500 tapes were in use in thirty-nine states and four foreign countries. One half of these were sold to hospice programs. In Bloomington, a group of local funeral homes purchased one for every school. And in April 1992, international education fraternity Phi Delta Kappa began offering the program to members through its Innovative Products Department. A sequel to the video, available in fall 1993, will offer schools a support curriculum based on Bloomington's *Griefbusters* after-school program.

A PROGRAM SURVEY

Today's programs come in a range of forms, from comprehensive kindergarten-through-grade-12 curricula with on-site training workshops, to train-the-trainer models that provide educators with materials plus the system of professional support necessary to conduct a program that meets their needs. Condensed support group and facilitator manuals offer less expensive alternatives and provide practical session formats and activities that are suitable for a variety of classroom, guidance, and after-school activities. Finally, several innovative programs make creative use of media such as puppetry, children's literature, and audio and video cassettes.

The following survey was compiled to illustrate several prepared, children's grief and loss programs available for use by hospice, school, and other professional staffs who work with children. Most, in fact, were developed by hospice professionals or those with previous hospice experience. They represent a range of approaches for application in classroom instruction, facilitator training, and support group formation in both school or after-school settings. This is not meant to be an inclusive list, nor a critical review; it is merely a sampling of options available. Information about the programs is based on input provided by program managers, participants, and literature. Inclusion of a program does not imply endorsement. Prices (1992) are included.

Programs are grouped into three categories. *Comprehensive* programs are those that are most intensive and provide the largest assortment of materials and resources for both student instruction and facilitator training. Although approach varies, they tend to emphasize on-site facilitator training and follow-up support. By the nature of their thoroughness, they often require the greatest commitment of resources and time.

Facilitative programs are a collection of training manuals, workbooks, and videotapes that provide professionals with some of the basic knowledge required to initiate a school loss program or activity. They either offer a source of program materials or recommend ways that facilitators can begin to assess those needs. They are an inexpensive and practical way for professionals to begin to address grief needs at school.

Creative programs explore concepts of grief and loss through a child's imagination, using puppet shows, children's books, audio-visual materials, or some combination of these. Whether presented alone or in conjunction with other programs or activities, these represent the most novel approaches to the subject.

There are also many supplementary activity books, films, and other resources that are available for educators. Some of these are listed in the Appendix under *Additional Resources*. Also included there are organizations that offer resources of their own. Again, space limitation does not permit an inclusive list.

Comprehensive

Children and Grief: Living with Loss
Created by Jessica M. Gurvit, M.A., 1984
Living with Loss, Inc.
P.O. Box 50399
Jacksonville, FL 32240-0399
(904) 241-2182
Fees: basic—$600 per school (minimum 25 schools),
       plus expenses

This intensive two-day workshop and training program for school systems was developed at Hospice of Northeast Florida, Jacksonville. The program operates under a facilitator model whereby teachers, volunteers, and counselors are trained to identify grieving children and provide them with information, coping skills, and the emotional support they need to overcome negative effects of loss. Training initially focuses on increasing awareness of school personnel regarding grief's impact on children, helps professionals differentiate between "healthy" and "unhealthy" behaviors, and suggests counseling intervention techniques to help children resolve their loss. The program also outlines evaluation and follow-up procedures and provides criteria for determining when additional professional counseling is recommended. The basic fee includes a preliminary needs assessment, training of administrative personnel, two-day training for three counselors per school, a training and resource manual for each counselor, and follow-up. Efficacy data is available for this award-winning program.

The Good Grief Program
Founded by Sandra Sutherland Fox, Ph.D., ACSW, 1983
Judge Baker Children's Center
295 Longwood Avenue
Boston, MA 02115
(617) 232-8390
Fees: based on hourly rate of $100–$200,
         plus travel expenses

Perhaps the first program of its kind, The Good Grief Program provides crisis intervention to schools and community groups when a child is terminally ill or dies. Among program services are crisis intervention; consultation to teachers, administrators, group leaders, and parents; in-service training for school staffs; educational programs for interested groups; and distribution of a variety of resource materials. The program's philosophy of children and grief is based on *Good Grief: Helping Groups of Children When a Friend Dies*, in which the late Dr. Sandra Fox explores the concept of "good" grief as involving four "tasks": understanding, grieving, commemorating, and going on. (The book is available separately and is included in the section on *Facilitative* programs.) In addition to its other services, the program maintains a resource library for use by participating groups and assists them in enlisting financial support to ensure continuation and success of the program.

Growing Through Grief
A K–12 Curriculum to Help Young People Through All Kinds of Loss
Donna O'Toole
Mountain Rainbow Publications, 2nd Edition, 1991
477 Hannah Branch Road
Burnsville, NC 28714
(704) 675-5909
Loose-leaf Binder: 392 pages, $59.95

This is an award-winning, comprehensive, general-loss curriculum that provides a life-skills approach to learning about loss. Separated into age groupings, the program actually provides three curricula: K–3, 4–8, and 9–12. Introductory chapters thoroughly explain how children understand grief and loss, and how adults can help them. These chapters include *The Importance of Grief in the Early Years; Recognizing and Understanding Losses of Young People; Developmental Issues; Understanding the Grief Process;* and *Helping Children Grow Through Loss*. Each unit in the curriculum has defined learning objectives and flexible formats that incorporate examples from literature and popular culture. Also included are more than 100 reproducible handouts, annotated resources grouped by age and needs, and units addressing death and suicide as special types of loss. Facilitator support is also available through tailored workshops.

Rainbows for All (God's) Children
Founded by Suzy Yehl Marta, 1983
Rainbows For All God's Children, Inc.
1111 Tower Road
Schaumburg, IL 60173
(708) 310-1880
Fee: $700, inclusive of materials and services for:
    Grades Pre-K–8, 30 participants, or
    Grades 9–12, 50 participants

An internationally recognized program, Rainbows for All (God's) Children offers comprehensive curricula and training for peer support groups of children, adolescents, and adults who are grieving a death, divorce, or painful family transition. Religious and secular versions are offered to schools, churches, and other community organizations in order to furnish students with an understanding of the grief experience, opportunities for emotional healing, a stronger sense of self-esteem, and coping techniques to help them transfer the pain of loss into personal growth. The programs are formated into 12 weekly sessions, plus wrap-up days, that use physical or writing activities, workbooks, storybooks, games, discussion, sharing, and reflection to explore grief feelings and experiences. The program requires one site coordinator and four to six facilitators. Training, as well as local, on-site facilitator support, is provided. The program can also help with additional resources as needed. Curricula for single parents and college-age adults are also available.

Facilitative

Bereavement Support Group Program for Children
Beth Haasl, B.S., and Jean Marnocha, M.S.W.
Bellin Hospice Program, Green Bay, WI
Accelerated Development Inc., Publishers, 1990
3400 Kilgore Avenue
Muncie, IN 47304
(317) 284-7511, (800) 222-1166
Leader Manual: 95 pages, $12.95
Workbook: 39 pages, $6.95

This is a five-session support group program for bereaved children, presented with a leader manual and participant workbook. Sessions are entitled *Introduction and Discussion of Death/Grief; Feelings/Self Esteem;*

Memories; Funeral Process; and *Coping with Grief/Wrap-up.* In addition
to the basics in children's grief reactions and caregiver techniques, the leader
manual covers nuts-and-bolts topics such as session outlines, group size
and location, number of facilitators, necessary time commitment, and even
includes sample brochures, letters, and invitations. The participant workbook provides worksheets and reading lists for each session. Special group
activities include a memory mural, puppet show, and storytelling and
writing.

Good Grief: Helping Groups of Children When a Friend Dies
Sandra Sutherland Fox, Ph.D., ACSW
The New England Association for the Education of Young Children
Boston: 2nd Edition, 1988
Distributed by The Good Grief Program
Judge Baker Children's Center
295 Longwood Avenue
Boston, MA 02115
(617) 232-8390
Book: 74 pages, $10

This practical, informative book serves as the basis for The Good Grief
Program, which is included in the *Comprehensive* program section. It introduces the concept of "good" grief and its four components: understanding,
grieving, commemorating, and going on. Chapters include *Children and
Death: What Do We Know?; Tasks for Bereaved Children; How Adults
Can Help; Vulnerable or Troubled Children;* and *Ideas in Action: Vignettes
of Interventions.* A guide to suggested resources—including films, books,
and articles—is also provided.

What Do I Tell My Children?
Leslie Kussmann
Aquarius Productions, 1992
31 Martin Rd.
Wellesley, MA 02181
(617) 237-0608
Video Cassette, 31 minutes, $150, $50 preview
Discussion Guide, 4 pages, $25 per 50

Joanne Woodward narrates this award-winning documentary recommended for professionals and families. The video is broken into five segments, based on Sandra Fox's model of "good" grief. Children and adults
talk about their experiences with death, and professionals then offer their
perspectives to viewers. A brief guide follows the video format to facilitate
group discussions. Segments include *Learning to Help Ourselves, Learning*

to Help Our Children, Understanding, Grieving, Commemorating, and *Going On.* Resources and support groups are listed.

When Grief Comes to School
Carol Ebeling, Ed.S. and David G. Ebeling, Ed.D.
Bloomington Educational Enterprises, 1991
P.O. Box 2178
Bloomington, IN 47402
(812) 332-0546 or (800) 489-9933
Video Workshop Kit, $69, includes:
Video Cassette, 69 minutes
Leader's Guide, 20 pages

This video program offers four separate presentations on grief and loss for an audience of school professionals. Concepts of the grief process, crisis intervention and planning, family needs, and bereavement are incorporated into a series of interviews with a bereaved student, a bereaved mother, a school principal, and faculty members. The leader's guide follows the video format, providing discussion suggestions and reproducible handouts. Total time allotted per session is suggested at 30 to 45 minutes. Facilitator support can be arranged in some cases, and consultation with local hospices or other professionals is encouraged.

Creative

Aarvy Aardvark Finds Hope
Donna O'Toole
Illustrated by Kore Loy McWhirter
Rainbow Connection, 1988
477 Hannah Branch Road
Burnsville, NC 28714
(704) 675-5909
Storybook: 80 pages, $10.95
Audio Cassette: 60 minutes, $10.95
Teaching Guide: 28 pages, $5.95

This is an illustrated, read-aloud book and audio tape that introduces the concept of loss through the story of an aardvark who is abandoned when his family is taken to the zoo. The story explores the roles of time, curiosity, metaphor, support, remembrance, and commemoration toward the goal of personal growth. The teaching guide explains how to teach grief concepts to children and gives suggestions for incorporating artistic expression into the learning process.

The Kids on the Block!
Created by Barbara Aiello, 1977
9385-C Gerwig Lane
Colombia, MD 21046
(800) 368-KIDS
Pediatric Hospice Program: $3,100

This internationally renowned, award-winning program uses life-size puppets to teach children about disabilities and differences. Characters and
skits address different issues and stimulate discussions after the show. Their
program on pediatric hospice was developed in collaboration with the U.S.
Office of Maternal and Child Health and Children's Hospice International
and features five characters: a terminally ill child, his brother, his hospice
nurse, a classmate, and his dog. The characters interact in four skits to
demonstrate to child and adult audiences the hospice care concept and how
a child, his family, and friends can learn to deal positively with terminal
illness, death, and bereavement. The cost of this program package includes
five life-size puppet characters, scripts, audio cassettes, props, a mini-
curriculum, and a comprehensive resource list. Programs are also offered
on topics such as cancer, AIDS, divorce, and a wide variety of disabilities
and social issues. *The Kids on the Block!* has its own series of materials,
including books, instructional resources, a video cassette, and puppeteer
training workshops.

The Death of a Friend:
Helping Children Cope with Grief and Loss
Susan Linn
New Dimension Films
85895 Lorane Highway
Eugene, OR 97405
(503) 484-7125
Film: 15 minutes, $320
Video: 15 minutes, $280
Rental: $32

This filmed puppet presentation was developed by The Good Grief Program at the Judge Baker Children's Center, Boston, as a way to help groups
of children begin to talk about the death or terminal illness of a friend. The
story line explores the fantasies and fears experienced by two friends when
a third friend is struck by a car and killed. It is designed for children from
preschool through the early elementary years, and it is also a good resource
for teachers and other adults who work with young children. A discussion
guide is included with each video that provides information about children's

understanding of death and dying, ways to use the video, suggested discussion questions, and a bibliography.

NOTES

1. Feifel, H. (1977). Death and dying in modern America. Death Education 1: 5–14.

2. Waas, H., Miller, M.D., Thornton, G. (1990). Death education and grief/ suicide intervention in the public schools. Death Studies 14:253–268.

3. Bordewich, F.M. (1988). Mortal fears. The Atlantic 261:30–34.

4. Kastenbaum, R. (1982). New fantasies in the American death system. Death Education 6:155–166.

5. Pine, V.R. (1986). The age of maturity for death education: a socio-historical portrait of the era 1976–1985. Death Studies 10:209–231.

6. Pine, V.R. (1977). A socio-historical portrait of death education. Death Education 1:57–84.

7. Kastenbaum, R. (1977). We covered death today. Death Education 1:85–92.

8. Crase, D. (1989). Development opportunities for teachers of death education. The Clearing House 62:387–390.

9. Levin, S. (1988). Lessons in death. The Dallas Morning Press, 17 April, 1F–2F.

10. Cullinan, A.L. (1990). Teachers' death anxiety, ability to cope with death, and perceived ability to aid bereaved students. Death Studies 14:147–160.

11. Rosenthal, N.R. (1978). Teaching educators to deal with death. Death Education 2:293–306.

12. Pratt, C.C., Hare, J., Wright, C. (1980). Death and dying in early childhood education: are educators prepared? Education 107:279–286.

13. Kübler-Ross, E. (1969). On Death and Dying. New York: Macmillan.

14. Fredlund, D.J. (1977). Children and death from the school setting viewpoint. Journal of School Health 47:533–537.

15. Wass, H. (1983). Death education in the home and at school. ERIC (ED 233–253):11–15.

16. Thompson, C.L. (ed.), Brookshire, M., Noland, M.P. (1985). Teaching children about death. Elementary School Guidance and Counseling 20:74–79.

17. Yarber, W.L. (1977). Where's Johnny today? Health Education 8:25–26.

18. Kaplan, D.M., Smith A., Grobstein, R. (1974). School management of the seriously ill child. Journal of School Health 44:250–254.

19. Zwartjes, G.M., Zwartjes, W.J., Spilka, B. (1981). Students with cancer. Today's Education 70:18–23.

20. Ross, J.W., Scarvalone, S.A. (1982). Facilitating the pediatric cancer patient's return to school. Social Work 27:256–261.

21. Ross, J.W. (1984). Resolving nonmedical obstacles to successful school reentry for children with cancer. Journal of School Health 59:84–86.

22. Overbeck, B., Overbeck, J. (1990). Helping Children Cope with Loss. Dallas: The Grief Resource Foundation, pp 9–2, 9–3.

10

Role of the Primary Physician

DORIS A. HOWELL

THE EVOLVING IDENTITY OF THE PRIMARY PHYSICIAN

In the last half century the practice of medicine and the role played by the physician have undergone major changes, moving from a predominantly simplistic art-science delivered in the home by family-oriented generalists to today's sophisticated office or hospital-based specialities. This change has been reflected in the preferential selection of the science scholar to study medicine. The growing size and sophistication of the science base demand students be able to acquire finely honed knowledge and skills with which to practice the complex diagnostic and therapeutic modalities of modern medicine.

The limited number of accredited medical school entry slots mandates fierce competition among well-qualified peers. Only the best gain admission. After matriculation the tension continues to mount, as the clock, rather than a peer, becomes the chief competitor for the student faced with a massive amount of essential information to be assimilated in incredibly short hours. Such pressure promotes a "loner" behavior in the scholar, who, in the pursuit of excellence, concentrates on science and, subconsciously, may deepen his knowledge by narrowing the breadth of interests.

There has been a growing concern that since World War II the body of medical science has increased in geometric progression, leading to an increased demand for specialists, with a subsequent reduction in the number of graduates entering primary care practice.[1] Efforts over the last two decades to control escalating specialty growth tracks have led to increased family practice training programs and have encouraged primary or general training tracks within internal medicine and pediatrics.

Unlike the more focused "loner" specialist, the primary care generalist seeks a broader view of the whole person and his lifestyle, not only the

172

disease or complaint, and tries to encompass the entire family within the doctor-patient relationship. Countries with successful nationalized health services have charged the primary physician with the overall evaluation and care of the patient, and the responsibility to serve as the gatekeeper to specialty services when indicated. The potential loss of adequate numbers of patient-oriented generalists represents a serious threat to the more humanitarian style of medicine, so sorely needed by the severely or terminally ill patient.[2]

DICHOTOMY VERSUS DYAD

Pediatrics, like internal medicine, is in itself a specialty covering the full panoply of illnesses and diseases in children up to 21 years of age. Subspecialties have evolved over the past fifty years to address the more complex aspects of system diseases once fluid balance and replacement therapy, preventative immunizations, and antibiotics changed the mortality and morbidity statistics for childhood. The generalized pediatrician has become the leader in applied preventive medicine, with a major goal to promote wellness and set the stage for a healthy life-style.[3]

Although certified as being well-trained in all aspects of the problems of childhood, the pediatrician is the first to admit that his specialty associates provide assistance in complicated or difficult situations where greater expertise is needed.

The more serious the condition or complicated the treatment, the greater likelihood that the sick child will be referred to or the parents will elect to see a specialist. When this happens, the dependency of the family on the expertise of the specialist can distance them from their primary caregiver unless the specialist clearly delineates the limits of his involvement and identifies the primary care physician as a collaborator and partner in the case. In turn, the generalist must become fully informed and assert himself as a partner with the specialist, in addition to the usual role as physician, counselor, and ombudsman to the child and the family.

Collaborative care does not come easily to the physician, whether he is a generalist or specialist. Through collaboration, attention to the needs and concerns of the patient are doubled; the specialist, freed from some of the routine care, gains time to serve more patients needing his expertise, while the primary physician sustains the strong bond with the patient and family on a regular basis. This cooperative alliance takes time, effort, and trust, but the benefits to the patient are significant.

In the care of children, the pediatric primary caregiver gains his first experience in collaboration by acquiring the confidence and trust of both child and parents. Although the physician must develop a bond with the child, it cannot be totally exclusive of the parents—the legal and rightful guardians. The measure of a successful relationship is evident when all parties are comfortable with the situation. One of the real rewards of primary care pediatrics is this special bonding with child and family that permits the pediatrician to play an integral role in the life of the child-patient. Sharing such a patient with another professional, even an expert, is not spontaneous, but demands a certain generosity of spirit. In admitting the need for greater expertise, the primary pediatrician must relinquish a major part of his autonomy and authority.

In most illnesses, the primary pediatrician may expect the return of the patient to his care with recommendations or treatment guidelines appropriate to the ongoing care. The specialist at that point steps back and assumes the role of pure consultant. In the case of serious or life-threatening illness, the necessary continuing presence of the expert may displace the primary physician as the child's medical guru. Some primary physicians, uncomfortable in handling serious illness or unwilling to mount the ongoing care of the high-risk child, may prefer to abrogate all care to the specialist. In turn, the specialist may feel that the severity of the condition requires his special care for all matters and bypasses the primary physician. The parents may feel that they must cleave to the specialist as the sole hope for the survival of their child and become uncertain or ill at ease in continuing their relationship with the referring primary physician.

In many geographic areas, the primary physician is not a pediatrician with three years or more of pediatric training, but a generalist who, having trained in family medicine, may feel less prepared to cope with the changing or sophisticated treatment regimens.[4] By intent or by default, the patient often becomes the primary responsibility of the specialist or is shared with several specialists for whom the first order of business is the cutting edge of science of the disease and its treatment. This approach offers excellent and appropriate medical care to the seriously ill child, but can be less than satisfactory to the patient and family if the specialist is too busy to communicate or bond with them or if distance from the specialist hinders continuity of care.

The talents and skills of multiple caregivers are essential in the development of a collaborative care plan. Anticipating the many needs of the patient over time in the expected course of a serious illness will facilitate the assignment of roles and responsibilities to the professional most able to respond in a timely and appropriate manner. Such a care plan will require frequent revision as the patient's course deteriorates and the concentration of care shifts from the treatment mode to one of increasing palliation and support.[5]

THE INTERPLAY OF ROLES

The most effective and holistic treatment for the terminally ill child requires that both the primary care physician and the specialist know their respective roles.

The Primary Care Physician

The physician who has been the child's primary health caregiver must be capable of being the case manager, freeing the specialist to serve as the authority during acute or critical periods and as the strategist for the therapeutic plan. The case manager needs to be cognizant of all aspects of the child's growth and development, her pattern of health, personality, and behavior. Likewise, he has a special bond with the family—both parents and siblings.[6] The primary care physician is most likely to know the family's religious ties, marital stability, economic pressures, and their sources of strength and support. As a practitioner in the community, he is knowledgeable about the available support resources and how to access them. He may also have a good working relationship with the school system, which will be invaluable in maintaining the school-age child's normal pattern of life for as long as possible. His availability to the family on a day-to-day basis, even if not exercised daily, provides a sense of security by maintaining continuity of care and by reinforcing pertinent medical information, decisions, and expectations. Many of his roles are shared with or performed by professional nursing, social work, and office associates, whose specific skills may exceed his own.[7]

Not all primary care physicians feel confident to assume this heavy responsibility because of either currently overextended schedules, distance from the designated specialist, or discomfort with the new or sophisticated therapies recommended by the specialist. Although in the best interest of the patient, it cannot be assumed that every primary care physician will be willing to take on a collaborative partnership in the continuing care of the patient. The willingness of the primary care physician to play an active role throughout the illness acts as a catalyst to promote collaborative interrelationships. When the primary care physician abrogates total care of the child to even a respected specialist, the family may feel abandoned, and the primary physician, himself, displaced and useless. In optimal care of child and family, a strong collegial relationship must develop between the primary and specialty physicians that allows a bond of trust to grow between patient, family, and physicians.

The Specialist

Many years of concentrated training are invested to prepare a physician with expertise in one definitive field of knowledge and skill. Patients are usually referred by generalists or other specialists because of this training and the specialist's demonstrated ability. In most treatable conditions, the specialist serves as consultant to the primary physician and, after a period of service, will return the patient to the original caregiver.

In the case of life-threatening illness, the need for the most expert knowledge is paramount. The specialist, to whom the child has been referred, cannot separate the disease from the child or the child from the family. He must establish an immediate rapport with the child and family with whom he has had no previous relationship. During treatment of the child's most acute phase of an illness, the specialist must assume leadership and prescribe the priorities in order to obtain optimal results. There are many periods in the semiacute, chronic, or deteriorating stages of illness that the maintenance of the child's condition may be more appropriately tended to by the primary care physician, freeing up precious time for the specialist to address those patients with acute or more sophisticated problems. Determining the ideal balance of care between the caregivers is very difficult, with the interplay of constantly changing variables affecting the outcome.

If the specialist has not maintained a close relationship with the primary physician during early stages of the child's illness, he may not have the benefit of the support of the primary physician in the terminal stage. Alternatively, the dedicated specialist should not desert his patient when the disease reaches the terminal stage. The patient and family need to appreciate that the combination of generalist and specialist can provide them with greater care and continuity of services. In contrast, when there is not a collaborative relationship the patient stands to lose, particularly if the primary physician feels excluded, withdraws from playing an active role, or is openly antagonistic. Logistically, the specialist cannot be all things to every patient, even with the help of a large support team, and the primary physician is not trained to meet the needs of every patient alone. Together, however, they make a powerful team.

RESPONSIBILITIES OF THE PRIMARY PHYSICIAN

The primary physician has numerous responsibilities when caring for the dying child including supervising the child's overall health, providing psychosocial care, and participating in case-management activities.

Overall Health Supervision

The primary physician, concerned with the total care of the child and not only the illness or disease, is mindful that each child should live as normally as possible, however long life may last. Furthermore, new advances in molecular medicine and genetic engineering, which might alter the deterioration, can only benefit the patient who has been maintained at the best possible level of general health and function.[8]

Children suffering life-threatening illnesses are not exempt from superimposed infectious diseases or accidents, although because of their serious underlying illness, they may even be more vulnerable. Prevention provides the best protection against intercurrent insults, which requires the primary physician to maintain constant surveillance for potential infection in the family, friends, school, and community.

All patients, regardless of prognosis, need prompt and appropriate treatment for infections and trauma so that the quality of life is sustained at the highest possible level. Immunizations need to be kept current, with highly specific ones for hepatitis and pneumococcus used to protect the immunocompromised or high-risk child.

Maintaining adequate nutrition presents a constant challenge in the terminally ill. The child may be nauseated, anorectic, or show a capricious appetite that bewilders the parents, seeking to please their child at any cost. The primary care physician, concerned about maintaining good nutrition, must find an equitable compromise. Only near the end of life does good nutrition become nonrelevant, when it is more appropriate to provide food and fluid purely for the comfort or pleasure of the child.

Psychosocial Care for Child and Family

A preexisting relationship with the child and the parents provides a strong foundation to support a family throughout a life-threatening illness. Never is it more valuable than at the time of diagnosis, when the family is shocked and unbelieving, and again in the terminal stage when grief and suffering turn to mourning. The behaviors of all family members impact heavily on the child and must be mobilized into supportive and comforting influences through anticipatory guidance directed by a known and trusted physician. The primary physician is also in a position to observe the family dynamics and identify persons, particularly siblings, who may not be coping well and who may need special intervention or assistance. The patient and siblings, often unable to verbalize their fears, can be helped through their suffering by the primary physician who recognizes and interprets acting out behavior and helps create outlets for the patient and siblings.

After the death of the child, the primary physician remains a pillar of support as he continues anticipatory guidance to the siblings, providing health supervision and preventive care while assuring himself and the parents that the grieving process is progressing normally toward healing. The primary physician is in a position to recognize the first signs of pathologic grieving in any family member. Even without special mental health training he may often need to assume the initial role of counselor-psychologist to distraught family members before referring them for specialized care.[9]

Case Management Responsibility

Should the primary physician elect to relinquish most of the care of the patient to the broader experience of the specialist, within the family he will still be looked to as counselor and friend to provide an overview of the case, to be able to translate and interpret for the parents new or unclear medical information and changes in the child's condition, to identify their rights and duties, and to validate the ongoing care. To function in this diplomatic role, the physician needs to have kept in close communication with the specialist and his staff about every change in the care of the patient. Concurrence among all caregivers will lend added support to the stability of the family through this stressful period.

The primary physician plays the pivotal role of facilitator to mobilize community resources for the patient and family should they choose to maintain the child at home, providing palliation with the help of community support. These community resources are so varied in quantity and quality that the primary physician must be well-acquainted with local options and the current availability of services to accommodate the needs of the child and family.[10]

Increasing numbers of children's hospitals and large pediatric services have developed an extension of hospital-based services to include a home care team. Such extended programs are likely to sustain the specialist in charge of all care, with the primary physician more remote. Specialists, with their broader experience in the field, tend to be more "cure oriented" and less ready to move from curative therapy to caring and supportive modalities. In children with cancer, the parents, as well as the specialist, may be reluctant to relinquish active therapeutic measures. When, ultimately, there is concurrence to move to palliative care, the primary care physician can be instrumental in orchestrating the supportive, comfort care in the child's home. All caregivers must be united in their efforts to comply with the child's wishes to be at home. Hospice home care or a local home health agency can provide professional and volunteer staff in conjunction with the physician to meet the needs of the entire family.[11] Hospice facilities providing residential care for children are relatively uncommon, except in Great Britain, where they have been of particular benefit in offering support and respite to the children with serious congenital defects and long-term neurodegenerative diseases.[12]

Hospice care in the United States has been identified uniformly with terminal care rather than palliation for long-term or chronic illness, with federal medical care reimbursement tied to less than six months of estimated survival. In children, illnesses needing palliation are often of a prolonged and chronic nature requiring specialized services and trained, experienced staff.[13]

Regardless of the locus of the terminal care, one physician needs to supervise and coordinate the services. In the child's best interest, the specialist, the primary physician, and the parents should decide, in advance, who will fill that role at each stage of the illness. The need for continuity of care across the entire continuum of illness requires constant adjusting and fine-tuning of services and personnel so that the patient and family can adjust gradually to the impending outcome without abrupt changes in caregivers or location. The primary physician should have the knowledge and ability to sustain the continuity of care, but can only be effective and at ease with such responsibility if he has maintained a close and fully informed relationship with the patient, family, and specialist throughout the entire course of the illness.

THE MOVE TOWARD THE IDEAL

The decade of the 1990s will see major changes in health care delivery systems. With growing impatience, U.S. citizens have been demanding a louder voice and a more central role in their own medical care. Recognition of the importance of prevention and the responsibility of the individual to exercise one's personal prerogative to be an active participant in one's own care is paramount in the person-oriented practices of primary physicians.

Public education, achieved largely through television and the media, has enhanced consumer knowledge of health and medicine, and citizens have become more vocal in questioning medical practitioners and challenging their paternalism. There has been a growing distress with perceived prolongation of life by physicians reluctant to let "nature take its course," particularly when the patient may not be relieved from suffering. The steadily rising cost of medical care has not been accompanied by clear evidence that patients' voices are heard or their needs addressed. The more affluent the patient the more frantic the pursuit of "cure," with diminished or absent attention to adequate palliation, psychologic or spiritual support. This perceived commercialism may be the final straw in the public rejection of the physician as trusted counselor.

Medical education, inundated by ever-expanding science, has been unable to free time from an overextended curriculum in diagnostic and therapeutic medicine, to promote training in the art of medicine—that is, in the care of the person, particularly in palliative and terminal care.[14,15] Modern technology has honed clinical diagnostic tools and skills, but communication and psychosocial skills are assumed to be intuitive and not in need of teaching.[16] These critical elements of the patient-doctor relationship are mainstays of primary care practice and should be essential tools in specialty practice. Many surveys of medical students and recent graduates attest that today's physician has been poorly prepared for practice in chronic and terminal illness, pain and symptom control, and medical ethics.[17,18] These studies have shown physicians' discomfort with and ineptness in issues of dying, death, and bereavement. Pioneer medical curricula at Case Western Reserve, McMaster, and Harvard Universities have sought to keep abreast of society's changing mores by preparing physicians with experience for gaining skills in all aspects of human illness: physical, psychologic, social, and spiritual; however, such programs are still the exception.

As we race toward the end of the twentieth century and look back at our successes and failures it is evident that the price of the emphasis on science and technology has been at the expense of the humanitarian core of the doctor-patient relationship. Increasing numbers of scholarly scientists and humanistic visionaries have voiced their concerns and recommendations in so compelling a manner as to survive editorial annihilation, and are prodding the medical profession to make the science of medicine fully responsive to human needs.[16]

In his teaching and writings over the past decade, Eric Cassell has stressed the discomfort of society at large in dealing with the personhood of interaction, particularly in medicine and most of all in the area of the physician's nemesis—terminal care.[19,16] Although medical education has been slow to respond, the inevitable need for change has gained momentum and will not be halted. The new breed of physician will restore the relief of suffering and concern for the person to the practice of medicine, making the profession whole again.

The primary care physician may find himself at ease with this changing medical milieu, more than the specialist or the educator, because the patient's needs have always been the major focus of his professional commitment. With this experience the primary practitioner should be able to play a leadership role in returning humanistic concerns to the practice of medicine.

In addition to a holistic approach to patient care, the primary physician's role as gatekeeper of the health-care system will influence not only the access to specialists, to secondary and tertiary care, but also to the distribution of scarce resources.[20] In addition to the medical and management skills one must acquire, familiarity with bioethical issues will be critical to this new role. Not all primary care practitioners will have had the preparation and training commensurate with the demands of such decision making and the weight of the judgment calls that will fall to them.[21]

The optimal palliation of the patient whose life is nearly at a close constitutes a major commitment from the physician. Although the primary care physician rarely perceived himself as a researcher, the definitive data needed on which to base treatment decisions in palliative care can only be derived from studies of the patient—his or her symptoms, coping skills, attitudes, quality of life, function, and suffering. Since palliative care has only been accepted as a specialty in the United Kingdom in the past two years, palliative practice has had little opportunity to be subjected to the rigor demanded of clinical research. The interest in palliative care by allopathic medicine has been limited primarily to anesthesiologists concerned with pain research. The hospice literature has documented many case reports and testimonials, but well-documented methodologic studies are needed to validate the effectiveness of palliation. Primary care physicians committed to relief of suffering for incurably ill patients need to base their care on well-researched clinical phenomena by using evaluative research tools with which to document observations of their patients. If palliative care is ever to be accepted as standard care, it must be shown to be credible, measurable, replicable, and scientific or it will be rejected by medical colleagues as emotionalism. Well-designed studies of the clinical practice of palliative care by primary physicians in the trenches can prove Derek Doyle's admonition: "Science and compassion are not incompatible."[22]

The primary care physician must also prepare himself for unknown new responsibilities, as has been demonstrated over the last decade with the explosive increase in patients suffering from Alzheimer's disease and AIDS. The pediatric primary practitioner may be spared the tragedy of Alzheimer degeneration, but AIDS is an iceberg of unknowns in the infant and child, with only the tip of the devastating disease and its complications visible. The intensity and style of palliative care that will be needed at various ages will become evident only through critically evaluated and documented clinical experiences over time. At the present time, the demand for palliative care for this passively transferred, highly fatal disease in children surpasses expectations as well as resources.[23] Research data in health services must parallel the clinical research to substantiate the need for palliative services and to provide these children some modicum of quality of remaining life.[24] In time, AIDS may become a disease of the past, but be assured that new afflictions with similar challenges will be waiting in the wings. The primary physician must prepare himself to deliver the same high-caliber care to those patients whom he cannot cure as to those he can.

The collaboration between specialist and primary care physician expressed in the preceding section of this chapter may have impressed the reader as idealistic and the concept as naive. Not so! There are many individual efforts at successful collaboration that speak to the realism of a professional dyad and the likelihood of success for collaborative care when the focus of care is on the needs of the patient. The changing model of tomorrow's physician from entrepreneur to Good Samaritan bodes well for patients and physicians alike.[25] The sophistication of modern medicine and future science advances cannot be applied to patient care except through embracing a collaborative health-care system.

NOTES

1. Aldridge, D. (1987). A team approach to terminal care: personal implications for general practitioners. J. Royal College of General Practitioners 37:364.

2. Colwell, J.M. (1988). Primary care education: a shortage of positions and applicants. Family Med. 20:250–54.

3. Lovejoy, F.H. and D.G. Nathan (1992). Careers chosen by graduates of a major pediatric residency program 1974–1986. Acad. Med. 67:272–74.

4. Byock, I.R. (1984). Hospice and the family physician. J. Family Practice 18:781–84.

5. Kohler, J.A. and M. Radford (1985). Terminal care for children dying of cancer: quantity and quality of life. Br. Med. J. 291:115–16.

6. Fernbach, D.J. (1985). The role of the family physician in the care of the child with cancer. CA-A Cancer J. for Clinicians 35:258–70.

7. Hill, F. (1990). Palliative care in the young. The Practitioner 234:292–96.

8. Howell, D.A. and I.M. Martinson (1989). Evaluation of palliative care: steps to quality assurance? Palliative Med. 3:267–74.

9. Behnke, J., E. Setzer, and P. Mehta (1984). Death counseling and psychosocial support by physicians concerning dying children. J. Med. Ed. 59:906–08.

10. Corr, C.A. and D.M. Corr (1985). Hospice approaches to pediatric care. C.A. Corr and D.M. Corr (eds.), New York: Springer.

11. Lauer, M.E., R.K. Mulhern, R.G. Hoffmann, and B.M. Camitta (1986). Utilization of hospice/home care in pediatric oncology. Cancer Nursing 9:102–07.

12. Burne, S.R., F. Dominica, and J. D. Baum (1984). Helen House—a hospice for children: analysis of the first year. Br. Med. J. 289:1665–68.

13. Corr, C.A. and D.M. Corr (1985). Pediatric hospice care. Pediatrics 76:774–80.

14. Buchanan, J., R. Millership, J. Zalcberg, J. Milne, A. Zimet, and I. Haines (1990). Medical education in palliative care. Med. J. Australia 152:27–29.

15. Bulkin, W. and H. Lukashok (1991). Training physicians to care for the dying. Am. J. Hospice & Palliative Care. March/April:10–15.

16. Cassell, E.J. (1991). The nature of suffering and the goals of medicine. E.J. Cassell (ed.), New York: Oxford University Press.

17. Benton, T.F. (1988). Medical undergraduates. Palliative Med. 2:139–42.

18. Murray, J.L., S.A. Wartman, and A.G. Swanson (1992). A national, interdisciplinary consortium of primary care organizations to promote the education of generalist physicians. Acad. Med. 67:8–11.

19. Cassell, E.J. (1982). The nature of suffering and the goals of medicine. N. Engl. J. Med. 306:635–45.

20. Gordon, A.K. (1989). The physician gatekeeper: access to the medicare hospice benefit. Am. J. Hospice Care, Sep/Oct:44–47.

21. Zaner, R. (1988). Ethics and the clinical encounter. Englewood Cliffs, N.J.: Prentice Hall.

22. Doyle, D. (1990). Facing the 1990's: special issues. Hospice Update. 2:1–11.

23. Daily, A.A. (1991). Terminal care for the child with AIDS. In P.A. Pizzo and C.M. Wilfert (eds.), Pediatric AIDS: The challenge of HIV infection in infants, children, and adolescents. Baltimore, MD: Williams & Wilkins, pp. 619–29.

24. McCormick, K.A. (1991). Future data needs for quality of care monitoring, DRG considerations, reimbursement and outcome measurement. Image: J. Nursing Scholarship. 23(Spring):29–32.

25. McDermott, W. (1977). Evaluating the physician and his technology. J. Am. Acad. Arts & Science (Daedalus) 106:135–57.

11

Staff Support

BERNICE CATHERINE HARPER

Caring for children is a challenge. Caring for sick children is a double challenge. Caring for dying children is an immense challenge. As a general rule, health-care professionals are trained to cure and to focus on living children, children getting well, children going home to their parents or significant others. This chapter's focus is on helping pediatric health professionals maximize their potential and talents in caring for dying children as well as preserving themselves and avoiding the burnout syndrome; living well mentally and psychologically with a strong administrative underpinning and support system. In other words, there must be job satisfaction and personal rewards for choosing to work in a pediatric setting with seriously ill and dying children. Caring has nothing to do with sentimentality because at the core of health-care services provided to seriously ill and dying children is the question: *How does one genuinely care, giving oneself totally yet preserving oneself totally?*

STAFF SUPPORT IN A THERAPEUTIC ENVIRONMENT

Hospitals and other health-care facilities as a general rule have not met the needs of dying patients, nor the needs of the health-care professionals who work with them. With a conscious effort and appropriate program planning in these facilities, the requirements of the administrators, physicians, nurses, social workers, occupational and physical therapists, speech and hearing specialists, chaplains, volunteers, and other health-care workers involved in the care of terminally ill children and families could be met. From the standpoint of the health-care facility, this approach will involve the development of a dynamic personal care system because it is not unusual for the total staff to mourn and grieve for a dying child. The dynamics of behavior must be understood and accepted by the staff of the health-care facility and the supervisory system, with the full and complete knowledge that this is an appropriate reaction during or after the death of a child.

Health-care training prepares health-care professionals to be helpful, skillful, and competent, but with dying patients their own emotions are exposed during the adaption and adjustment process. A major question is how does one go about developing that all-important ego-strength that is indispensable in the integration process that is needed to be comfortable with the dying patient and the family? This building seems to be dependent on the health-care professional having supervisors on whom they can model and pattern-set.

A Major Role for Supervisors

The supervisor must have an understanding and an acceptance of the fact that until the health-care professional has come to grips with his or her own feelings about death and dying, it might be hard to love a dying child. Supervisors must comprehend the grieving process that health-care workers must go through if they are to be effective in working with dying children and families.

The supervisor must also appreciate the emotional impact dying patients have on the staff who must work with them. The supervisor must be supportive, understanding, and accepting of workers as they undergo the experiential growth sequence, without being inappropriately judgmental of the professional's emotional reactions. In addition, the supervisor must be able to tolerate the various aspects of the professional's behavior without internalizing, and use his or her knowledge to first help prepare the professional for the experience and to lead the professional through the emotional adjustment process. The supervisor must also know about the growth experiential process and have worked through his or her own feelings about life's end and the in-between process before he or she can give help and support to staff.

Finally, the supervisor needs to distinguish between appropriate and inappropriate behavior, such as forgetfulness when caused by an overwhelming situation, or not coming to a conference or being late for staff meetings. The degree of anxiety and emotional trauma exhibited by health professionals must be brought into balance in proportion to the overall situation.

The willingness on the part of the health professional to share his or her feelings about working with a dying patient will provide an avenue of release for pent-up emotions and tensions, and free the health professional to experience a positive growth process. A strong supportive, health professional–supervisor relationship is necessary.

Awareness of Needs

Professionals can help patients die with dignity only if they feel dignity and self-respect in their practice and with the supervisor. The professional must see those who have been successful and who practice with dignity, respect, calmness, determination, and dedication.

All health workers must be aware of the needs of dying patients, their families, and other health professionals. However, all health professionals cannot and should not be encouraged to work with dying patients. There should be self-selection and self-election with a joint health professional–supervisor assessment of the individual's capacity to perform and achieve some gratification and job satisfaction. On the other hand, it is important that no health professional be the only one who works with the dying patient and the family, which has tended to be the practice in some facilities. Caring for a dying child must be a *shared* professional experience and responsibility involving the departments, organization, and other staff, as the burden is too great for any one person to carry or shoulder.

Terminal illness and death represent trauma that brings forth deep emotional anxieties for the professional. In the helping process, the health-care professional needs to (1) understand the dynamics of behavior of the patients who will not recover; (2) relate to the actions and reactions of the relatives; (3) give care, counseling, support, and strength to the patients and members of the family; and (4) understand and deal with their own feelings and anxieties.

Caring versus Curing

Knudson and Natterson believe that the professional composition of the staff is important; that a high degree of interprofessional cooperation is required; and that the importance of a stable professional population cannot be overemphasized.[1] Health professionals who work with dying children are confronted with several problems. Foremost is the fact that the satisfaction of curing an illness will not be available, in contrast to other patients. Health professionals must have the capacity to deal constantly with apprehensive, demanding, and depressed patients and families. "To die is the human condition. To live decently and die appropriately and well is man's privilege and needs to be one goal of service among helping professionals."[2] According to Kjellstrand, "Physicians need to teach themselves to recognize better the shadow line between prolonging life and prolonging dying and to understand that death should be a human act of dignity and not a prolonged mechanical failure that can be fixed with even more technology."[3]

The Facility as a Support System

Support for the health-care professional is required from the health-care delivery system, the supervisory staff, the community, and the person-patient-family system. All of these systems impact on each other. As Rozett points out,

> Institutions already deeply involved in rendering services to the dying and their families must acknowledge their responsibility by openly establishing a value system for the care of the dying, and by creating lines of responsibility or accountability to implement the level of humane care needed in the field. This means institutions should present information about dying in their in-service training programs. It means encouraging staff members to discuss their personal problems with and their different viewpoints about coping with dying patients, and it means providing staff members with a structured opportunity to grieve and look inward following the death of a patient. Staff members, too, we must remember, need support and an opportunity to ventilate when confronted with death.[4]

Working with terminally ill and dying children is a unique work experience requiring specialized skills, adaptation and adjustment, coming to grips with death, dying, and the in-between life processes, and decision making.

FRAMEWORK FOR STAFF SUPPORT

Health-care professionals must go through an adaptation process in order to become comfortable in working with patients who are facing death and dying. This growth process has been visualized along the line of a "Comfort-ability Scale"[5] (Figure 11.1). This scale represents the stages of growth and development, involving cycles of productive change, observable behavior, and feelings. It can be said that the steps on the model represent the narrative sequence of emotional and psychologic progress made at each stage. This growth is reflected as the health-care professional gains understanding, knowledge, and strength, and works through conflicts, internal and external, thus adding a new human caring dimension to one's existing capacity to be helpful. In other words, this deep compassion is the maturing of the health-care professional. In Figure 11.2, the stages reflect one purpose of this model, which is to look at the growth of cognitive development in relation to the coping mechanism in a stressful, traumatic situation, and thus avoid burnout.

The underlying assumptions for such a model are that (1) the human personality develops according to steps predetermined in the growing person's readiness to be driven forward, to be aware of, and to interact with a

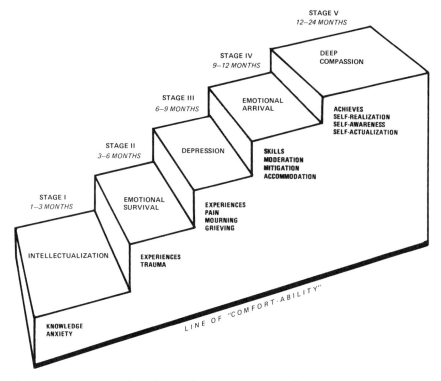

Figure 11.1 Coping with professional anxiety in terminal illness. (Source: Harper [5]).

widening social radius; and (2) society tends to be constituted to meet and invite this succession of potentialities for interaction and to safeguard and encourage the proper rate and the proper sequence of their unfolding. Erikson refers to this as the "maintenance of the human world."[6] Health-care professionals do not enter practice academically, intellectually, or emotionally prepared to deal with death and dying. They must learn to cope with their anxieties arising from their caregiving experience. This process requires an adjustment period for them, a time for adaptation and working through their feelings about death, dying, and the in-between life processes. Health-care professionals should not be left to suffer in pain psychologically as they work with seriously ill and dying children and their families. Professional anxieties in catastrophic diseases and terminal illness are observable phenomena for which a coping mechanism can be developed.[5]

Stage I: Intellectualization

It is important to understand how the health-care professional can confront his or her own anxieties about death. The Comfort-ability Scale illustrates the five stages of coping with professional anxieties in terminal illness.

The health-care professional in Stage I is anxious about death; death is threatening to the personhood. It is also known as the stage of intellectualization and may occur during the first three months of working with terminally ill children. Contributions to the children and families are mostly in the area of physical care and tangible services, without investigation of in-depth feelings. Baths have to be given, children have to be fed, medications have to be administered, examinations have to performed, and blood has to be drawn. X-rays must be taken, back rubs given, dressings changed, and occupational and physical therapy procedures carried out. Other contributions include participating in therapy, looking at drawings and pictures, handling social work activities and pastoral visits and taking care of admission and discharge procedures. In other words, staff confronts death on an intellectual basis through use of knowledge, facts, and medical and social procedures.

Health-care professionals in Stage I have to become familiar with the health-care setting: hospital, hospice, home, special childrens' units, and other facilities. Professionals working with a terminally ill child are exposed to a two-pronged threat because they must become familiar not only with the health-care facility, but also with the physical disease and the dying and death of children. In hospice care there is a need for an adaptation and adjustment period in order to become comfortable in assisting terminally ill children and their parents.

Consider the following excerpts from supervisory conferences.

Vague, nebulous expressions are all I contain within me after three months in my work. It is not that I am unfeeling, but my feelings as they exist now are a conglomerate mixture without organization.

Mrs. G. came in the ambulance with her son when he was brought to the hospital for the first time. She had only learned of the diagnosis of leukemia that morning. She met me with the words, "Why my son? I've always taken good care of him. He's my only son and I can't have any more children."

I had looked at the trembling woman in front of me—her eyes brimming with tears. I felt uneasy as I considered the total situation. That evening my thoughts kept darting back to Mrs. G. and her critically ill son.

Stage II: Emotional Survival

During Stage II, the health-care professional may experience trauma, frustration, and sadness. Trauma is experienced in the area of the psyche, which causes an emotional reaction as the health-care professional begins to relate to the reality of the dying child. The health-care professional may feel frustration when he or she realizes that the child is going to die and that the health-care team, no matter how superior, cannot prevent the

Stage I	Stage II	Stage III	Stage IV	Stage V
Professional knowledge	Increasing professional knowledge	Deepening professional knowledge	Acceptance of professional knowledge	Refining of professional knowledge
Intellectualization	Less intellectualization	Decreasing intellectualization	Normal intellectualization	Refining intellectual base
Anxiety	Emotional survival	Depression	Emotional arrival	Deep compassion
Some uncomfortableness	Increasing uncomfortableness	Decreasing uncomfortableness	Increasing comfortableness	Increased comfortableness
Agreeableness	Guilt	Pain	Moderation	Self-realization
Withdrawal	Frustration	Mourning	Mitigation	Self-awareness
Superficial acceptance	Sadness	Grieving	Accommodation	Self-actualization
Providing tangible services	Initial emotional involvement	More emotional involvement	Ego mastery	Professional satisfaction
Utilization of emotional energy on understanding the setting	Increasing emotional involvement	Over-identification with the patient	Coping with loss of relationship	Acceptance of death and loss
Familiarizing self with policies and procedures	Initial understanding of the magnitude of the area of practice	Exploration of own feelings about death	Freedom from concern about own death	Rewarding professional growth and development

Working with families rather than patients	Over-identification with the patient's situation	Facing own death	Developing strong ties with dying patients and families	Development ability to give of one's self
		Coming to grips with feelings about death	Development of ability to work with, on behalf of and for the dying patient	Human and professional assessment
			Development of professional competence	Constructive and appropriate activities
			Productivity and accomplishments	Development of feelings of dignity and self-respect
			Healthy interaction	Ability to give dignity and self-respect to dying patient
				Feeling of comfortableness in relation to self, patient, family, and the job

Figure 11.2 Stage characteristics and differences of the schematic growth and development scale.

death. Sadness is experienced when the health-care professional begins to cope with his or her own future situation and the realization that I, too, will die. Thus, the process of grieving for self and one's own mortality becomes an emotional issue.

Stage II, the survival stage can take place from the third- to sixth-month period. The following is an excerpt from a supervisory conference.

> This morning as I looked at Anna — those little chubby hands have wasted to a mere skeletal form, the long dark eyelashes that had formerly framed sparkling brown eyes now gone dull, the little legs so withered and drawn — something deep within me cried. I mourned because of the change from a beautiful baby to a slight whimpering human form. When leaving the room, the sorrow I felt changed to a venomous hate.

Stage III: Depression

Stage III involves further growth and pain, with depression being the most noticeable element of this stage. It is the most critical of all of the stages in the Schematic Growth and Development Scale for the health-care professional learning to cope with death and dying.

An individual will experience the impact of death in Stage III in different ways. Some health-care professionals may experience extreme anxiety, grief, and depression. They may question their usefulness and ability to contribute and be helpful, and also express anger, hurt, and self-doubt. Individuals may have an "inability to come to grips with the situation," a time for health-care professionals to "grow or go." In this period of growth, development, and experimental experience, mastery of one's self and feelings become a challenge. The health-care professional begins to accept death and its reality. Individuals in Stage III try to accept what they will do or shall do about working with terminally ill children. If they are still in the "shall" mode, then there is a possibility of those individuals leaving the job.

The "will" concept is needed for movement and is the forerunner for emotional advancement into the next stage. The timeframe of Stage III is from the sixth to the ninth month.

Here are additional excerpts from supervisory conferences:

> It is a bittersweet experience . . . this attraction, these children, and the pain when these brave little soldiers face separation from life. How can one stand by with a dry eye when he hears a 4-year-old telling the priest during last rites: "When I get to heaven, I'll bless you too," or an older child asking that he always be remembered. I feel drawn toward and pulled apart at the same time.

As I am immersed in this emotional experience, I find myself less in touch with reality. I ignore doing necessary dictation on expired cases.

I do the same tasks over twice. I absentmindedly forget an important appointment.

I see constantly the fine line between life and death. I repeatedly see parents whose eyes are welling with tears. I also see the effect on myself — the emotional exhaustion at the end of the workday.

The sources of strength increase, however, as quickly as the sources of stress. My personal religious faith affords such strength as does the following biblical text: "the Father of mercies, and the God of all comfort . . . comforteth as in all our tribulations, that we may be able to comfort them which are in any trouble, by the comfort wherewith we ourselves are comforted of God." (2 Corinthians 1:3–4)

Stage IV: Emotional Arrival

From the ninth to the twelfth month, Stage IV or Emotional Arrival is achieved. This stage is reflected by a sense of self-protection and productive behavior in taking care of the terminally ill child while coming to terms with internal feelings. There is moderation and mitigation in relation to the sense of loss and death; accommodation and ego mastery also take place.

The health-care professional can now feel like a helping human being and can participate in healthy interaction. Now the individual has the ability to work with and on behalf of the dying child. These activities and skills may or may not be new to the health-care professional, but he or she is now free from the constant and deep-seated emotional concern about his or her own death and dying. Knowledge, skills, and human-caring competencies can now surface and become observable through behavior and job performance. The learning, assimilating, emotional articulating, understanding, accepting, and adjusting of the mind and body have occurred. Health-care professionals no longer have a need to imagine or feel that they, too, may be suffering from the same illness as their patient. At this stage, there is a moving away from identification with the patient's symptomatology.

This emotional freedom in no way can make the health-care professional feel less concerned about their patient. They are now able to take hold and let go emotionally more easily. Their hurts are less frequent. Less time is required for getting over the deaths of their patients. These are important goals in the growth and development process or accommodation and ego mastery. They give impetus to the role, position, and professional stance that the health-care professional is now able to assume. The ego mastery occurs over fears, anxieties, trauma, grieving, and depression that may have blocked the health-care professional's ability to meet the needs of their dying patients and families. Another excerpt from a supervisory conference:

> In this sudden moment of retrospective thought, I realize there were differences between the first experience and now. I was not the same person I was 12 months earlier. A growing process, a molding of ideas, and an incorporation of experiences had taken place within me.

Stage V: Deep Compassion

Self-realization, self-awareness, and self-actualization are the components of this stage. All stages must be experienced before arriving at Stage V.

At this stage of growth health-care professionals have been involved with the care, treatment, and management of the disease. They now know and can understand and accept the fact that, in some cases, living can be more painful to the terminally ill child and family than dying.

Learning, growth, and self-development have taken place in Stage V through anxiety-producing trauma, pain, and depression. The result of this developmental process, however, has promoted professional growth and satisfaction. The health-care professional has now developed the ability to give of one's self to the terminally ill child. Behavior and performance are enhanced through dignity and self-respect.

The deep compassion felt by the health-care professional toward the terminally ill child is translated into constructive and appropriate activities based on a human and professional assessment of the needs of the patient, family, and significant others. Without the development of skills that results from passing through Stages III and IV, Stage V cannot be reached. This final stage is reached in one to two years. Consider the following excerpts from supervisory conferences.

> Yes, there are happy emotions. There is the satisfaction of successfully helping many families through the largest crisis they shall perhaps ever face.

> Extreme tiredness often comes over me. . . . This tiredness has a numbing effect on both sad and happy feelings.

> I feel privileged to have worked with this staff for whom I have found great respect. It is a staff where love is measured with the medication and caring mixed with the medical competence.

> I also feel a better person for this work experience. One's values change. I realize now that it's with people and ties with them that the importance of life is found.

BURNOUT AVOIDANCE STRATEGIES

The health-care professional's grief is quite different from that of the terminally ill child or surviving family members. Different adaptation, adjustment, and coping mechanisms are required. Ultimately, health-care professionals can cope with their grief and the professional anxieties that result from working with the dying child. Working through the aforementioned five stages will result in a commitment and dedication to serving a child who is dying, with love and without being afraid.

"Wordless comfort" must be present in all units, sections, facilities, and programs designed for dying children, their families, and staff. In other words, the emotional atmosphere must radiate love by actions, deeds, behavior, and performance. Staff members must show love, dignity, and self-respect in order to provide these caring attributes and activities to dying children and their families.

A background of love, warmth, caring, and sharing must be created. This will enable staff to feel the love for each other and to free staff members to give equally of themselves to their patients and families without undue depletion of themselves and their own caring capacities.

There are a wide variety of strategies that institutions can use to reduce burnout. An understanding of the grief process is critical to the success of supporting staff members.

1. The health-care facility must accommodate death work and reflect a quiet, active, and caring environment.

2. The administration, starting with the boards of directors, must have an understanding of the work to be done and must be supportive of the program; needs of terminally ill children and their families, and the importance of staff support.

3. Directors and supervisors must be role models for those professionals undertaking and commencing work with the terminally ill and dying either in hospitals, hospices, or home health agencies.

4. Supervisors must demonstrate an ability and a willingness to be involved. They must recognize that not all professionals may come to their practice prepared socially, emotionally, intellectually, and academically to work with dying children and their families.

5. Health-care professionals who desire to work with the terminally ill and dying must be able and willing to engage in a learning and developmental process.

6. All health-care professionals on a service unit must be aware of the

needs of dying children, their families, themselves, and other members of the staff. However, only the most knowledgeable health-care workers should be encouraged to work directly with dying patients. There should be self-selection and self-election together with a joint health-care professional–supervisor assessment of the individual's capacity to perform adequately and achieve job satisfaction. On the other hand, it is important that no health-care professional be the only one who works with the dying and the family. Such a burden of responsibility must be shared by many members of the department, organization, and institution.

7. Health-care professionals who experience personal death must be given appropriate time to adjust to these deaths with ample opportunities to do their own necessary grief work. If a professional is not given this opportunity to grieve, professional behavior may become cold and callous. Health-care professionals need recognition and acknowledgment of personal death, someone to talk or share feelings with, someone to cry with, or a shoulder to lean on. Grief treats become important: an apple, a piece of candy, kind words, a hug, an invitation to lunch, or any activity that shows caring, understanding, and empathy. Health professionals need what family members need, if they are to be free to remain caring and productive staff members.

8. All health-care professionals will require respite from the daily burden of working with the dying child and the family. This allowance must be built into the health-care facility, its program, be it a hospital, hospice, special unit, or home care agency.

9. Institutions must acknowledge that working with dying patients and their families is a traumatic experience of varying degrees for the health-care professional. Anxiety of varying types is believed to be inherent in those working with dying patients and their families. However, excessive anxiety is a disorganized and a destructive agent with regard to healthy adaptation.

10. Educational programs must be continuous and on-going with the topic of emotional involvement included in the curriculum. Several variables are thought to be beneficial to the adjustment of health-care professionals working with dying patients and their families: (1) the health-care professional's desire to be helpful; (2) the orientation and understanding of the diagnosis, illness, and prognosis; (3) the health-care professional–supervisory relationship; (4) the support system of the primary unit; and (5) the overall hospital environment and milieu.

A Dynamic Future

Being a health-care professional in the decade of the 1990s is a hard job— "more with less and less and less." But health-care professionals must continue to acquire a greater understanding of the political process; recognize and deal with the changing nature of hospitals and other health-care institutions; help to shape their futures, relative to the care of terminally ill children and their families; and help lay out the strategy for using that power to empower themselves.

The time is ripe for the renewed interest in the areas of staff support and hospice care for children. While we have come to accept the high technology and space-age breakthroughs of our culture, we still need to apply that knowledge and our energies on our health-care institutions. In addition, we are increasingly called on to address the moral issues of the distribution and access to health care. These challenges will not be overcome by technical advances alone. For the dying child, or for any patient, there is no substitute for the care that is provided by qualified and dedicated health-care staff.

NOTES

1. Knudson, A. and J. Natterson (1960). Practice of pediatrics: participation of parents in the hospital care of fatally ill children. Pediatrics 26:482–490.
2. Feifel, H. (1973). The Meaning of Dying in the American Society, Dealing With Death. University of Southern California at Los Angeles: Ethel Percy Andrus Gerontology Center, p. 7.
3. Kjellstrand, C. (1992). Who Should Decide About Your Death? JAMA 267: 103–104.
4. Rozett, R.T. (1973). Some Basic Principles of Death and Dying, Workshop on Death and Dying. State of Connecticut, p. 18.
5. Harper, B.C. (1977). Death: The coping mechanism of the health professional. Greenville, SC: Southeastern University Press.
6. Erikson, E. (1963). Childhood and society. New York: W.W. Norton.

12

The Volunteer Component

PAUL R. BRENNER

It is my assumption that there will be three different kinds of readers of this chapter:

1. Persons from hospice programs already serving adult patients who are considering extending their services to include pediatric patients and who are interested in how their existing volunteer component needs to be expanded to accommodate this special population.
2. Persons from organizations who are interested in establishing pediatric hospice programs, having no or very limited programs of direct volunteer services already in place, and are looking for "how to do it" information.
3. Persons from existing hospice programs that serve children and have operating volunteer services and are interested in reviewing their program of volunteer services.

In order to address such a wide diversity of interest and experience, this chapter will seek to present basic as well as comprehensive information about the service and management issues involved in establishing and maintaining an effective program of volunteer services to serve pediatric hospice patients. Different readers may, therefore, find it helpful to use the chapter headings to identify topics most relevant to their needs and interests, while others may benefit from reading the chapter as a whole.

VOLUNTEER SERVICES ARE REQUIRED

The Medicare and Medicaid benefits require that "the hospice documents and maintains a volunteer staff sufficient to provide administrative or direct patient care in an amount that at a minimum, equals five percent of the total patient care hours of all paid hospice employees and contract staff."[1]

In addition to adhering to the federal requirements, states which have licensure laws regulating hospices will need to review the specific requirements concerning the volunteer components in their state's regulations. As of 1990 these states include: Arizona, Alaska, Colorado, Delaware, Florida, Illinois, Kentucky, Louisiana, Maryland, North Carolina, North Dakota, Nevada, New York, Ohio, Oklahoma, Oregon, South Carolina, Virginia, Washington, Wisconsin, West Virginia, and Wyoming.

In the Definition of Children's Hospice Care adopted by Children's Hospice International, trained volunteer services are mandated, along with medical, nursing, psychosocial, and spiritual care services, as part of the continuum of care.[2]

THE VALUE OF VOLUNTEERS

There are three different perspectives on the value of volunteers: the perspective of the recipients of services, the perspective of the institutional provider, and the perspective of the community.

Traditionally, health-care providers like hospitals have not used volunteers to provide direct services to patients, but have used them in ancillary activities to services, such as distributing favors or magazines to patients, providing directions, or other kinds of facility-specific information to visitors. As the hospice movement evolved, however, it placed volunteers into a unique direct service role with patients and their family members. (Throughout this chapter the term *family* is used to describe any relationship of significance to the patient, not just blood relatives or marriage relationships.) As such, volunteers within the hospice system of care are considered to be unpaid staff.

In the hospice movement it is recognized from the beginning that the complex and varying needs and problems of the terminally ill and their families were of such a range that even skilled professionals could not address them all appropriately. Lay volunteers do not confront the same role expectations that confront a nurse, chaplain, social worker, or therapist. By being free of those role expectations, volunteers are receptive to information that patients and family members believe would not be important to a professional, but may be of significance for effective management of the case.

In addition, volunteers can provide much needed respite care to family members, by permitting them time away from the patient with confidence that the patients will be in the hands of someone who understands what is happening and is competent to respond to needs or problems that may arise. Simply by providing family members the opportunity to shop, to take care of other business, or to just get away and do something enjoyable, enormously enhances the ability of the family to manage the demands of caring for someone who is seriously and chronically ill.

However, the value of volunteers is not only measured by the dimension they add to a interdisciplinary care system for patients and family members, but also their implications for the role of the community.

The general withdrawal of social support for people with terminal illnesses has been well-documented in the so-called death and dying literature.[3] Volunteers from the community provide a way for members of the community to bring needed social supports to persons who may be experiencing withdrawal or abandonment from their traditional system of supports. The hospice volunteer institutionalizes a way for the community to continue to be involved and make a positive difference in the lives of its vulnerable members.

Finally, of course, volunteers also represent a certain cost-effectiveness for the total care. The Hospice Medicare legislation required that hospices demonstrate "the cost savings achieved through the use of volunteers,"[1] by documenting the positions that are occupied by volunteers, the worktime spent by volunteers in those positions, and an estimate of the dollar costs of that time saving.

PEDIATRIC HOSPICE CARE IN CONTRAST TO TOTAL HOSPICE CARE

According to statistics gathered by the National Hospice Organization in its 1990 survey of 1743 hospice providers, 95% reported criteria which allowed for the admission of children while only 67% actually had a pediatric admission. Of the 206,684 patients admitted nationwide in 1990, less than 1%, or approximately 2400 were children.[4] There is no available information on how many hospice providers have a specific pediatric program of hospice care in comparison with providers that include children without distinct staffing, policies, and procedures which delineate the care.

A summary statement of the differences between hospice care for children and adults adopted by Children's Hospice International identified four major areas of differences between pediatric and adult hospice care.[5]

First, the patients differ in the following ways:

1. These children are not legally competent to make their own decisions regarding medical services.
2. They are in a developmental process that affects both their under-

standing of and ability to articulate concepts of illness and health, life and death, loss and grief, and God and spiritual meaning.

3. They have not yet achieved a full and complete life and realized their life potential.
4. They may not have the verbal skills to articulate and describe their personal needs and feelings.
5. They will frequently protect parents and other significant persons at personal expense to themselves.
6. They are often cared for in a highly technical medical environment.

Second, the family issues of these children differ from the families of adult patients in the following ways:

1. These families may contain other minor children who are siblings to the patient, and there are often difficulties in communicating with them, involving them in care, and maintaining normal family patterns.
2. They tend to fear that the patient-child cannot be cared for as well at home as in the hospital.
3. The grandparents experience helplessness in dealing with their own children, the parents of the sick children, and the other grandchildren, and they grieve the loss of the continuity of the family.
4. These families tend to be under the stress of care and the burden of the child's disease for an ever-increasing period of time as treatments become more successful in extending time of life, increasing the need for respite care.
5. They tend to have less reimbursement options available to them and more financial strain.
6. They are under pressure to do everything possible without consideration in the attempt to save the child at any cost.
7. They tend to need to protect the child from information about the status of the disease.

Third, the issues which impact on the caregivers, the physicians, nurses, social workers, chaplains, who serve the patients and their families, differ in the following ways:

1. Caregivers tend to need to protect children, parents, siblings, and all others from the truth of what is happening.
2. They have a sense of failure in not being able to save the child, regardless of what they do.
3. Caregivers tend to have a strong sense of ownership of the child, sometimes to the exclusion of the parents, and may even assume they know best what the child needs.

4. They may have out-of-date concepts about pain management for children, especially infants.
5. Caregivers may have "unfinished business" relating to dying and death that may affect the style of care and what decisions are made for treatment options.
6. They may not be sensitive to the developmental stage of children or their cognitive levels.
7. Caregivers may not be fully informed about the processes of children's diseases.

Fourth, there are issues which impact on the institution or agency:

1. There is usually limited reimbursement for the services that are needed, and additional funding must be secured.
2. There is usually a high-staff intensity in caring for these children at home.
3. There is a need for special competencies in order to manage issues such as developmental levels, family-sibling issues, and pain assessment.
4. There is a need for a different focus on bereavement care.
5. There may be strong resistance by physicians to make a six-month terminal prognosis.

All of these differences have implications for the ways volunteers are recruited, screened, trained, assigned, supervised, supported, evaluated, and recognized.

In the next section, these differences will be delineated within a comprehensive outline of the framework of a volunteer component in a hospice program serving children.

STANDARDS FOR THE VOLUNTEER COMPONENT
OF A PEDIATRIC HOSPICE

In the evolution of hospice care for adults, standards have been developed at the state and national levels to provide a systematic, comprehensive way to organize and manage care. Some of these standards are incorporated into licensure laws and certification processes. Some, like the standards developed by the National Hospice Organization and Joint Commission On Accreditation of Healthcare Organizations, are voluntary and have attempted to move beyond the minimum levels often required by law.

The following is the author's attempt to put these various sets of standards into one framework that may be of value to persons who are organizing and managing a volunteer program for the first time, or persons who are already managing existing programs. In general:

1. The volunteer program shall be an organized program with written policies and procedures for all aspects of the program: recruitment, screening, training, assignment, supervision, evaluation, continuing education, support, discipline, recognition, and budget.
2. Volunteers shall be treated as staff members who are unpaid, which means they shall be managed in a professional manner and work with a written job description, policies, and procedures.
3. Volunteers shall have rights that are written and disseminated, including a grievance procedure.
4. The volunteer program shall be directed and coordinated by a designated person responsible for the program, who shall have a designated supervisor and written job description.
5. The hospice shall have a mechanism to ensure that an adequate, comprehensive, and appropriate written evaluation of the volunteer program is done at least on an annual basis.
6. The volunteer program shall be included in the equal opportunity, antidiscrimination, and confidentiality policies of the hospice.
7. The volunteer program shall maintain an adequate number of volunteers to respond to the need for volunteer services by patients and family members.
8. The volunteer program of services shall be integrated into the ongoing program of clinical services through equal participation in the activity of the interdisciplinary care team.
9. The volunteer program shall have a budget adequate to manage and support the services it provides.

MANAGEMENT OF A VOLUNTEER PROGRAM

The leadership of the volunteer program is critical to its success. The person responsible for managing the volunteer program frequently coordinates the largest number of individuals serving the hospice program, therefore requiring both organizational and managerial skills, as well as significant and effective interpersonal skills.

In the managerial role, the Coordinator of Volunteer Services needs to be able to accomplish at least the following:

1. Maintain adequate and up-to-date personnel files on each volunteer.
2. Maintain an up-to-date list of available volunteers.
3. Schedule needed volunteer activities such as training, in-service education, and recognition events.
4. Maintain regular communication with volunteers through mechanisms such as newsletters, memos, meetings, and phone contacts.

5. Ensure appropriateness, accuracy, and timeliness of documentation of services by volunteers.
6. Create and monitor a budget for volunteer services to ensure adequacy of materials and support activities.
7. Ensure that the volunteer services of the hospice receive appropriate and adequate public relations coverage.
8. Organize effective outreach programs to recruit appropriate volunteers.
9. Provide written reports to the supervisor about the accomplishments and needs of the program, including all required statistical information concerning visits, services, and hours of activity.
10. Provide mechanisms for improvement of the volunteer program.
11. Provide for inclusion of appropriate gender, age, racial, cultural, ethnic, social, and religious diversity in the volunteer program.
12. Organize and run effective meetings.
13. Assist the hospice program to utilize its volunteers creatively, effectively, efficiently, and appropriately.

In the interpersonal role, the Coordinator of Volunteer Services needs, at least, the following characteristics and abilities:

1. An interest in and enjoyment of people, since creating a mutual relationship with volunteers is important to the success of the program.
2. Good listening skills to identify not so obvious feelings, problems, and needs of the volunteers.
3. Effective supportive skills to provide empowerment, encouragement, and affirmation of the volunteers and their activities.
4. Crisis intervention skills to deal with volunteers' problems when they arise and the ability to resolve the situation in the most satisfactory manner.
5. Verbal skills to communicate with volunteers clearly, nonthreateningly, and nonjudgmentally.
6. Interpretive skills to define and articulate the unique role of volunteers in the delivery of services with the professional members of the hospice team and with the community in general.

Managing a well-organized and effective program of volunteer services is a challenging job. The *a priori* to all the managerial and interpersonal skills is the need for the person coordinating the volunteer program to be well grounded in hospice values and practice. From this perspective the coordinator needs to embody both what hospice is about as well as possess the ability to articulate and demonstrate it effectively.

RECRUITMENT OF VOLUNTEERS

The recruitment program for volunteers is a targeted marketing outreach to connect the needs for volunteer services with appropriate candidates for training as volunteers.

The hospice needs to inform the potential volunteers as fully and clearly as possible about the need for services, the role and responsibilities of volunteers, how the volunteers will be trained, supported, and utilized, and the amount of time expected. The straightforward dealing with volunteers begins with recruitment, not afterward. Materials that seek to recruit volunteers need to be honest in how they represent the hospice and its program of volunteer services.

Outreach may be offered to previous families served by hospice; religious institutions, community, professional and service clubs and organizations; and community organizations with a commitment to or interest in the care of seriously ill children and their families.

The hospice may establish a policy of not enrolling a volunteer who has experienced the recent loss of a family member for a specific period of time following the death, to ensure that the person will not be adversely affected by an assignment that would interfere with the provision of needed and appropriate care to a family and patient.

Outreach may be done through newsletters, news releases, brochures, public service announcements, news stories, videos, presentations, and talk shows.

It is important that every effort be made to recruit volunteers who appropriately represent the constituency served by the hospice in terms of gender, age, race, religion, ethnic background, language, culture, and education. This is important because frequently the volunteer is experienced by patients and their families as the person within the service delivery team who is most like them or has the most in common with them. The more commonalities that can be experienced in the relationship, the more likely it is that the volunteer can play an effective and helpful role. At the same time, since this may not always be possible, the volunteers who are recruited need to be able to function comfortably and effectively within cultural diversity and other significant differences.

SCREENING

Standard practice in hospice programs is to screen potential volunteers before they enter the training program.

This screening provides an opportunity to assess motivation, ascertain unfinished business which may interfere with volunteer effectiveness, and identify special needs, priorities, concerns, specialized ability or expertise, previous experience with serious illness, dying, death and grief, availability, and personal expectations.

The purpose of screening is to determine, as well as possible, whether potential volunteers are appropriate or not to undertake volunteer responsibilities with children and their families. While some volunteers may be strongly motivated to want to do this work, there may be other considerations that may limit their ability to be effective. In this case the screening interview will help these persons assess more realistically what they need to be doing now, and when it may be better for them to consider volunteering with the hospice.

When persons are not deemed to be appropriate, this unsuitability needs to be carefully explained to the individual and possible alternatives for volunteer involvement recommended. As much as possible the reason needs to be presented "objectively," such as "Your loss is still quite recent, and we recommend at this time that you wait. Sometimes the volunteer has to deal with very stressful feelings and situations, and that may still be very difficult for you." In no way should the individual be treated as inferior or inadequate. It is important to document the interview.

For potential volunteers who may be appropriate for training, the screening interview provides an opportunity to meet with a person in the hospice organization, to begin to develop a relationship with the hospice, and to answer the first line of concerns about getting involved. Frequently, at this point, potential volunteers express concern whether they can handle the emotionality of the volunteer experience and wonder if they will have enough time to give. Through the interview process, a more realistic understanding of the role and its activity can begin to take shape.

It is important that the screening criteria be written, standardized, and used consistently with each potential volunteer. A written record of the screening interview needs to be put in the volunteer's personnel file.

There is also a way in which the training program itself is a screening process, as the trainees are confronted with actual case situations and the emotionality of care. If trainees are unable to manage the intensity of the training, that is a significant indicator that they may not be able to manage their role as a volunteer.

TRAINING

There is an interdependence between training, the provision of services, and the evaluation of services. Training prepares volunteers to deliver ser-

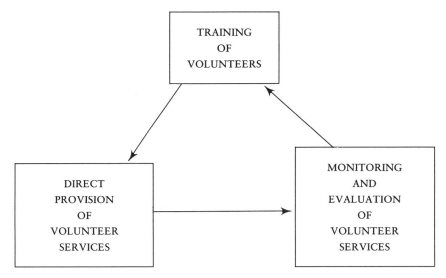

Figure 12.1 Interrelationship of the activities of hospice volunteers.

vices that meet the needs of children and their families. The volunteer services that are delivered directly are continually monitored and evaluated for their appropriateness and effectiveness. On the basis of what actually happens and what actually is needed, recommendations are made that can improve the effectiveness of the training program and meeting patient-family needs through volunteers.

The training program for volunteers shall be written with specific learning objectives and expected outcomes in terms of attitudes and values, skills, and behaviors.

Hospices which serve children and adults usually have a basic core of training that all volunteers are required to attend, and then a specialized core of additional training which relates specifically to pediatric care issues. Programs that serve only children can be specifically pediatric and do not need a specialized training component.

In staffing the training program, appropriate members of the various clinical services will be involved that the volunteers will be working with. However, it is most important to also have experienced volunteers participate as trainers as much as possible.

The distinctiveness of hospice care has been based on its commitment to specific attitudes, values, and principles, which need to be articulated in the training:

1. Dying and death as a normal part of life.
2. The right of the dying to have as qualitative an experience of life as possible all the way to the end.
3. The home as the preferred place of care for a terminally ill person.

4. Palliative or comfort-oriented care as the preferred kind of care for the terminally ill.
5. Inclusion of family members in the care provided, including at least one year of bereavement follow-up for family members after the death.
6. Provision of care for the terminally ill and their families through an interdisciplinary team within a comprehensive integrated system of home care, outpatient care, and inpatient care services.

At the same time, participants in the training program need to be provided adequate and enabling opportunities to explore their own attitudes and values about dying, death, loss, and grief, and those values of others that are different from their own.

In order to accomplish these learning objectives, the curriculum needs to incorporate experiential learning principles and approaches as much as possible.

The skills to be mastered by training participants include:

1. Use of key terminology, concepts, and characteristics of hospice philosophy, services, and history.
2. Ability to describe organizational structure of the hospice, its service delivery system, identify its key staff, and its basic finances.
3. Ability to describe the processes of dying and grieving and how to support them.
4. Ability to verbalize and conceptualize their own feelings, beliefs, and experiences with loss in an appropriate way.
5. Ability to articulate relevant cultural and spiritual differences surrounding dying and death.

The behaviors that are expected of volunteers after training include:

1. Effectiveness in fulfilling volunteer roles and responsibilities with patients and families.
2. Appropriateness in documenting services.
3. Participation in continuing education and support activities.

The structure of the curriculum will include both generic hospice items and specific pediatric items.

The generic hospice items included:

1. History of hospice movement.
2. Hospice philosophy of care.
3. Hospice interdisciplinary team management and services.
4. Palliative care.

5. Hospice levels of care.
6. Family systems theory, different types of families, dysfunctional families, impact of impending loss on families.
7. Loss, grief, and its characteristics and resolution.
8. Listening skills.
9. Crisis intervention.
10. Confidentiality regarding services and information.
11. Informed consent.
12. Documentation.
13. Role of volunteers.
14. Hospice grievance procedures for patients and volunteers.

While there may be appropriate pediatric references throughout the "generic" topics, the specific pediatric issues which need to be addressed, either as part of the above or separately, include:

1. Child and adolescent cognitive, psychosocial, and spiritual development.
2. Childhood illnesses, characteristics, and treatments.
3. Impact of ill children on families and family systems.
4. Nonverbal communication of and with children.
5. Special problems of home care for seriously ill children.
6. Relationships with other pediatric service providers.
7. Pain and symptom management of children.
8. Issues concerning the care of siblings of ill children.
9. Volunteer support in the inpatient setting.

Throughout the training it is important to monitor the participants and to note reactions, verbal skills, support skills, and other indicators of ability to be an effective volunteer. How a person responds and behaves may provide some valuable cues as to how that person will behave as a volunteer.

At the end of the training, a written evaluation tool of the training needs to be provided each participant, and the evaluations utilized to improve training. This evaluation is the first opportunity for the hospice to measure how successful it is in preparing volunteers for their role.

Upon completion of the training, each volunteer shall have had an accurate and confidential personnel file established containing all information initially required, which shall be secured and maintained in a confidential and protected manner.

Some programs may choose to schedule a second screening interview at this point.

Since a volunteer is considered an unpaid staff member, each volunteer will need to have at least a PPD (tuberculin) test annually, and a letter from a physician stating the person is free of disease that can be communicated casually and is able to serve in the role of a volunteer.

ASSIGNMENT

Every effort needs to be made to make the best possible match between volunteer and patient-family unit, if both are to have a mutually satisfactory experience.

It is incumbent on the person making the assignment to gather as much information about the patient-family as possible, as well as knowing the volunteer well enough to determine how effectively the relationship may work.

The volunteer shall receive an adequate orientation to each assignment by the Volunteer Coordinator. This information shall include at least:

1. Full name of patient and family members.
2. Accurate address with clear directions.
3. Accurate phone number and indication of best times to call.
4. Name of the primary nurse who will be the case manager and immediate supervisor and how to contact the nurse with problems.
5. Name and role of other staff members involved in the care and their role.
6. Identification of other agencies when involved in care.
7. Description of any needs, circumstances, special considerations, and identified problems.
8. Suggestions of what the volunteer's role may be.
9. Identification of case supervisor if different from primary nurse.
10. Identification of time, date, and place of interdisciplinary team meetings when there will be case review so that the volunteer can participate when possible.
11. Identification of whom to contact when there is an emergency, and how.

It is very helpful if there is an ongoing means of communication from the primary nurse who is managing the care, so that the volunteer has the experience of being treated as a full partner of the team, rather than an "appendix" to the paid professionals. Volunteers shall be informed routinely and in a timely manner of changes of status or levels of care of patients and their families.

Volunteers shall not be assigned to situations for which they are not qualified or prepared to respond or serve.

SUPERVISION AND EVALUATION

During the time the volunteers are assigned to a specific case, volunteers shall be clear as to who their supervisor is and to whom and how to submit their documentation. This supervisor shall be available to provide support and direction as needed throughout the course of the care.

There shall be an opportunity to evaluate the effectiveness of the volunteer's services on the written form for the evaluation of services filled out by patients and families. The results of this evaluation shall be shared, in an appropriate way, with the volunteer in order to improve services.

Volunteers shall be provided opportunities to evaluate the support and direction they received while on an assignment, as well as for the volunteer program in general.

At least, annually, an evaluation of each active volunteer shall be made, which shall become part of the personnel file.

The purpose of supervision is to assist the volunteer in every possible way to become more effective in the delivery of services, and therefore to feel more fulfilled as a volunteer.

Documentation shall also be included in the individual volunteer personnel file about assignments made and services provided.

Some hospices have found it very helpful to have a Volunteer Advisory Group, which serves as a liaison between the Coordinator of Volunteer Services and the corps of volunteers. Such a group can provide valuable input into the ongoing development and improvement of the volunteer program as well as serve as a problem-solving resource to the coordinator for assistance and help when needed. Such groups often meet quarterly and keep minutes of meetings regarding decisions made and actions taken. Members usually are active volunteers representing the various distinct volunteer service areas of the hospice, such as home care, inpatient care, bereavement, spiritual care, and special areas, such as puppetry and play.

CONTINUING EDUCATION

The hospice shall provide an organized continuing education program for its volunteers providing direct services to patients and their families. This program shall be planned with input from active volunteers or the Volunteer Advisory Group as well as other staff members who have working contact with volunteers.

Continuing education events shall be scheduled to facilitate the widest possible participation by all volunteers. Increasingly, as more volunteers are unavailable during traditional business hours, these events need to be planned for off work hours.

Participation in continuing education events shall be documented and included in each volunteer's personnel file, and each volunteer is expected to attend at least one such event a year.

It is also essential that the Volunteer Coordinator be given adequate opportunity for continuing education to increase job skills and effectiveness.

SUPPORT

Some hospices provide a mentoring program that assigns newly trained volunteers to experienced volunteers. New volunteers can accompany the veterans through their cases, or can have the veteran provide support through their first case.

In addition, hospices provide regular support meetings, which are especially designed to be helpful to newer volunteers.

In general, support will be offered to volunteers in a wide variety of ways:

1. One-on-one support in person and by phone through the supervisor or coordinator and a mentor.
2. Formal support meetings with a facilitator.
3. Notes or letters through the mail.
4. Contact by other members of the interdisciplinary team also involved in the case.

For the support program to be effective, volunteers need to play an active role in its planning and evaluation.

Some volunteers will also need much more support than others.

Many programs have a newsletter for the volunteers to keep them informed of hospice activities and opportunities for support and sharing.

DISCIPLINE

It is not always comfortable or easy to address inappropriate behaviors by volunteers. Nevertheless, it is important to address them as promptly and effectively as possible in order to correct the inappropriate behavior, lest patients and family members suffer adversely as a consequence.

It is imperative that volunteers are aware of the grievance procedure of the hospice to handle such problems when they arise, and that volunteers are subject to dismissal in the same way that paid staff is for actions such as sexual harassment, using drugs or drinking while on service, making prejudicial statements or judgments, violating confidentiality, breaking appointments without notice, and other inappropriate behaviors.

Volunteers need to know that they will have a fair hearing and may use the grievance procedure without fear of retaliation.

RECOGNITION

Although many volunteers fulfill their volunteer service with little or no need for recognition, there are also other volunteers who need a great deal of recognition for their service.

The hospice can provide informal ongoing recognition as services are provided, as well as some kind of annual formal recognition event. Some hospices have secured free meals at restaurants or other donated prizes for volunteers, while others provide recognition pins or other similar awards.

It is important that the contribution made by volunteers is reported to the community in as many ways as possible through newsletters, fact sheets, brochures, press releases, feature articles, talk show interviews, and presentations. The community needs to be made aware of the extraordinary service provided through the volunteers.

BUDGET

To provide an effective program of volunteer services, an adequate budget needs to be in place. This budget shall ensure that the following operational needs can be addressed appropriately:

1. Brochures or materials for volunteer recruitment.
2. Brochures or materials for volunteer services utilization.
3. Training materials and events.
4. Production and mailing of volunteer newsletter.
5. In-service and support events and materials.
6. Recognition activities and materials.
7. Books, videos, tapes, library and special training materials.

For a start-up program, the budget also needs to include:

1. Adequate office space for coordinator.
2. Appropriate office furniture.
3. Appropriate equipment, including computer work station.
4. Lockable cabinets for storing personnel files and other confidential materials.

ROLES

Volunteers in hospice are primarily used to provide direct services to patients and their families. Direct services can be defined in a variety of ways:

1. Volunteering in one's professional role.
2. Serving as a home care volunteer.
3. Serving as an inpatient care volunteer.
4. Serving as a special services provider with special expertise or training in spiritual care, bereavement care, AIDS, or some other skill.
5. Serving as a special activities volunteer, such as using puppets, pets, play, music, or art.

Volunteers, who may not feel comfortable being involved with providing direct services, are also needed. Indirect services include:

1. Clerical and other office support.
2. Help with fundraising.
3. Participation in speaker's bureau.
4. Preparation of volunteer newsletter or other newsletter.
5. Member of Advisory Group.
6. Serving as a member of the Board of Directors.
7. Other area of administrative expertise.

It is essential that nondirect service volunteers also be given a clear job description, be assigned a designated supervisor, and document their services and time.

SPECIAL CONSIDERATIONS

A few hospices have experimented with the use of children as volunteers, often through staff members who bring their own children along on visits. This can be very effective because the child "volunteer" will be perceived as a friend by the sick child.

When this is done, the hospice needs to have a consistent policy governing it. This policy needs to address the preparation of the child for the visit, discussion with the parents of the sick child, and a means of monitoring what happens.

Increasingly, high schools are requiring volunteer services from their students. Hospices may want to explore linking with local high schools to provide additional support for their children and adolescent patients and siblings of patients. Such a program will also have the effect of educating the students and the faculty about hospice care and the needs of the dying and the bereaved.

CONCLUSION

Volunteers have a crucial role to play in the provision of pediatric hospice services.

An effective volunteer program does not just happen. It is created and maintained with much work, not only from the coordinator of the program, but the entire staff and organization of the hospice, including the Board of Directors.

NOTES

1. State of Maryland (1991). Regulation 418.70(e), Standards 0555 and 0560. Home Health Agency and Hospice Regulations, Department of Health and Mental Hygiene, pp. 49, 50.

2. Children's Hospice International. Definition of Children's Hospice Care. Alexandria, VA, revision, July 7, 1989.

3. Kübler-Ross, Elisabeth (1978). To Live Until We Say Goodbye. Englewood Cliffs, NJ: Prentice-Hall.

4. National Hospice Organization, Arlington, VA. Information provided to author.

5. Children's Hospice International. Children's Hospice Care: Differences Between Hospice Care for Children and Adult Hospice Care. Alexandria, VA, August 27, 1989.

PART III

Appendix

An Early Model of Care

JULIE SIMPSON SLIGH

Edmarc Hospice for Children was created in 1978 as a ministry of a small church in rural southeast Virginia by a young couple whose own child, Marcus, was dying. Their efforts were supported by their pastor, Edward, who was also terminally ill. After the minister and the child died, the organization was named Edmarc to honor the memory of these two important people.

Edmarc has grown tremendously since that humble beginning and now serves a 2400-square-mile region incorporating eight cities, two counties, and a population of one million people. It has served 300 families and is presently following more than 100 families in bereavement. The average daily census is 45 families with a yearly census of 85 to 90. The agency provides a comprehensive package of clinical and family support services which are described here. It also serves as a training site for nursing and social work students as well as medical residents. As one of the only free-standing pediatric hospices in the country, Edmarc staff often act as consultants to other groups interested in providing pediatric hospice home care.

HISTORY AND DEVELOPMENT

For the first three years Edmarc Hospice for Children was funded by state grants to provide services to disabled and/or mentally retarded children. After three years the agency obtained a Certificate of Public Need for a home care hospice, which paved the way for licensure as a home health agency so that we could provide hands-on nursing care. In 1982, Edmarc received a private gift of $250,000 from the women of the Presbyterian Church, USA. That gift provided the funds to hire an Executive Director and to develop and expand the hospice services into the neighboring metropolitan region. It was enormously helpful to have the funds to deliver care as needed before we had the capacity to bill for services.

Once home health licensure and Medicare certification were obtained and money could be brought in through billing for services, more staff was gradually hired. Aside from an Executive Director, a secretary, and a part-time Family Services Coordinator, all of the permanent staff were nurses for the first five or six years. As the daily census reached 25 to 30, the agency had a full-time Director of Professional Services (who is a nurse), two full-time nursing supervisors, and a number of part-time nurses in the field.

For many years Edmarc was primarily a nursing agency. The social, emotional, and even spiritual support was often provided by its nursing staff. As the census grew and the financial base became more secure, ancillary services were added, such as physical therapy, occupational therapy, speech therapy, home health aide services, then medical social services. All of those services are eligible for reimbursement through health insurance. The noneligible services, such as bereavement care and volunteer coordination, came after seven to eight years of caring for families and hearing the general medical community and the agency's own field staff advocate for more comprehensive services. These comprehensive services are funded entirely through philanthropy.

PATIENT/FAMILY CHARACTERISTICS

When Edmarc first developed hospice admission criteria, using the adult hospice model, it expected to see children with cancer, children with less than six months to live, and patients seeking palliation but not cure. Staff quickly learned that such a patient profile rarely exists in pediatric hospice. Contrary to the adult hospice experience where a majority of the patients have cancer, only 35% of the pediatric patients had cancer. Unlike adult hospice patients whose life expectancy is usually less than six months, most of its children are admitted without reference to remaining life expectancy because physicians are usually not able to state that their pediatric patient has less than six months to live. Also unlike adults who can decide to stop further attempts at cure, we encountered parents who were unwilling to stop treatment even if there was only a slim chance of saving their child's life. Consequently, we have found it prudent not to restrict admission to patients who are expected to live less than six months and who are no longer seeking cure.

Furthermore, the agency learned that families with critically ill children who may or may not be labeled as "terminal" also need the total family care that a hospice uniquely offers. Children with progressive diseases, such as muscular dystrophy or advanced cystic fibrosis, in whom the course of the disease is definite but the life expectancy is unknown, are in families that are suffering many of the same stressful effects as those whose children have been labeled "terminal." The hospice philosophy is to look at the entire family rather than just the patient. Holism in hospice means that we address the needs of mind, body, and spirit: the social, emotional, physical, spiritual, and financial impact of the child's illness, from diagnosis to death and beyond. These factors are just as real in families with children who are likely to live another few years as in those who are likely to die very soon.

We have learned that many pediatric hospice patients who were expected to die, did not, and many who were expected to live a long time, died quickly. Edmarc's mission statement now states that it serves families with children *at risk of dying* in childhood. The practical interpretation of "risk of dying" includes admitting children as early as the time of diagnosis when their diagnosis carries a poor prognosis. For instance, we would be likely to admit a child with acute myelogenous leukemia at diagnosis, but a child with acute lymphocytic leukemia would probably be admitted only when he or she relapsed. We admit severely disabled children, such as those profoundly brain damaged following an accident, because those children statistically do not live into adulthood. We admit children with degenerative diseases, such as leukodystrophy, because they will almost surely die very young. We also admit children with congenital anomalies or genetic syndromes because they tend to have multiple system failures; we do not know how long they will live but we know they will not live long. Edmarc offers home health and hospice care so it avoids the potentially painful confrontation caused by a hospice referral. Instead, we tell parents that their child will be admitted for home health care and transferred to hospice if that need should arise. Historically, the distribution of diagnostic categories is as follows: 35% cancer, 25% cerebral impairment, 8% neuromuscular disease, 7% cardiac impairment, and 15% in other illnesses, including genetic disorders, accidents, and some rare conditions.

One of the important distinctions about pediatric hospice care is that the primary caregivers, the parents, are relatively young. Sixty percent of the patients are under 5 years old and most are in families where the parents are in their twenties or thirties. These families are usually not financially stable, so the uncovered medical costs quickly use up all of their resources. They typically have other young children who are forced to cope with difficult circumstances, which causes the parents great stress and guilt. Extended hospitalizations tear the family apart, leaving one parent to stay at the hospital and the other to maintain some stability at home. Siblings of the sick child become the forgotten grievers as parents necessarily devote their immediate attention to the dying or deceased child.

It is hospice's challenge to make this time endurable for pediatric hospice families. By helping to relieve daily stress, by lessening the guilt from "abandoning" other children, and by giving them the skills they need to care for their child at home, we help them to survive. Although we cannot cure the child, there is much that can be done to heal the family.

SERVICES

Skilled nursing care is offered on a per visit basis and private duty care on an hourly basis. The visits are done by registered nurses, the hourly care is done by licensed practical nurses. The amount of hourly care that is able to be provided is related to the physical needs of the patient and the amount of insurance coverage that is available. For patients with unskilled needs, they can be provided with a home health aide if the circumstances warrant that level of support.

Respite care is a fundamental need of many pediatric hospice families, especially those with long-term chronically ill children. Respite support is provided through nursing care in increments of at least four hours, so that the mother knows she can leave the house or take a nap if needed. The patient needs to qualify for nursing care, however, in order to be able to receive this type of service.

We have recently started a program funded through a private grant wherein we provide a home health aide for several hours at a time to those children not qualified for skilled nursing or we train a family friend or relative, at no cost to them or the family, to care for the child in the absence of the parents. The goal of this program is to build on the family's own support system. Many friends or relatives would babysit if they were not so intimidated by the child's physical needs. The Edmarc nurse trains them one-on-one until they feel comfortable enough to care for the child alone.

Many parents want to or must return to work and are in need of specialized care for the disabled or critically ill child. Some of the patients could live for five or six years in a debilitated state. The agency can only provide full-time care when full insurance reimbursement is available because this service is so expensive. Meeting this need is one of the constant challenges and frustrations.

Many of the hospice patients are severely disabled either because of their disease or their condition. Physical therapy (PT) is provided as a part of the team approach to enhancing quality of life because these services offer or increase comfort and may restore muscular function. PT also helps to keep the child flexible enough to be more easily handled by parents and to prevent further injury. Occupational therapy helps children, whose remaining life spans are unknown, to maintain dignity and functioning. Pediatric occupational therapists are also skilled in dealing with feeding problems common in these children. Speech therapists help children develop alternative modes of communication and are also a resource helping with oral feeding problems. One of our children lost speech as a result of his brain tumor—the speech therapist taught sign language to him and his family.

The medical social services are provided by a master's-level social worker. She does short-term counseling, family assessments, information-gathering and referral services, and funeral planning. She designs and staffs the sibling support groups and all social events for families. She facilitates spiritual support services by working with the families' own identified pastoral resources or by calling on Edmarc's clergy volunteers.

The bereavement care is provided by a full-time Bereavement Coordinator who is a bereaved mother whose own son was cared for in our hospice program. She leads the bereaved mothers' support groups and organizes the bereaved fathers' support group that is facilitated by a volunteer professional. For more than a decade, a bereavement consultant has worked with the agency, and helps with special bereavement events such as the annual Memorial Service and bereavement retreats.

The bereaved parents' retreats have been very successful. We borrow a vacation home near the shore and invite bereaved fathers and mothers to participate in a weekend of sharing. They are separated into groups that are facilitated by local mental health professional volunteers. This event is held as needed but usually twice a year.

The staff are also planning a bereaved families' camping weekend. It will take place from Friday evening through Sunday afternoon and will consist of therapeutic and age-appropriate activities for all family members. The goal is to improve communications and relations within bereaved families and to learn from other bereaved families' coping skills.

The volunteers do not work directly with the pediatric patients, except in rare cases when the patient is communicative and seeking companionship. Instead, the volunteers are used primarily for family support to parents and siblings and for help in fund-raising, office work, and as chaperones for sibling events.

We host an annual summer picnic for all current and bereaved families, staff, and volunteers. This event gives families a rare opportunity to socialize in a place where their special needs are understood and shared by others. At Christmas, volunteer caroling teams go to all Edmarc family homes bearing gifts for all family members. They also take a picture of Santa with the hospice child and family; photographs that are treasured by parents.

A Board/Staff planning retreat is held every year. It is unusual for organizations to have board and staff together for an all-day planning session, but it has been extremely successful. Most of the best ideas for creative programming have come out of this retreat.

STAFF

The agency uses two types of nurses. Pediatric nurses provide care for acutely ill children with skilled needs or for infants. For children with fewer skilled needs, good nurses are used, whether or not they have strong pediatric experience. Often a nurse's professional experience in adult hospice or personal experience with a terminally ill relative makes them an excellent candidate as a nurse for a family, especially if the child's physical needs are not highly technical and the patient is a little older.

Hospice nurses are trained in a variety of ways, depending on their individual experience. For the highly technically skilled pediatric nurses with no hospice experience, we provide in-service education on both hospice and corporate philosophy. For nurses with a background exclusively in adult care, in-service education focuses on the specific skills they will need for a specific child, for example, on the use of a new port-a-cath. Although nurses can be trained to enhance their professional skills, they cannot be trained to have the appropriate caring attitude; so personality counts heavily in Edmarc's hiring practices. Its experience has been that this work is attractive to a narrow segment of the nursing population so there is a lot of self-selection before they apply for a job.

In pediatric hospice, staff burnout is predictable and can be very rapid, reflected in a fairly high rate of turnover among nursing staff. In an effort to avert or postpone burnout, supervisors try to evenly distribute the emotional burden when possible. Permanent staff who have several patients each are mixed with those who moonlight on a case-by-case basis, taking one patient and family at a time. Edmarc has the distinct advantage of having a tertiary care pediatric hospital in the area from which it is able to attract part-time pediatric nurses. All of the nurses are hired with the expectation that they will stay with the family through the death or discharge of their patient. Remarkably, even in cases where the child has lived for many months or years, the majority of nurses have stayed through to the end of care. Some of these nurses started out with a once-weekly visit and stayed through the once- or twice-*daily* visit periods.

There is a trade-off between using one nurse for many patients and using many nurses who are moonlighting for one patient at a time. One nurse who has several patients will usually accept new cases, which enables the agency to admit a child and have a nurse immediately available. The problems arise when that one nurse has experienced a number of patient deaths. Burnout, leading to resignation, is always a risk. The nurses who moonlight and have only one hospice patient at a time "cost" time spent hiring and training but they usually are willing to give considerable extra time and attention to their hospice families. If they experience a death and decide not to work with hospice for a while, staffing capacity is only reduced by one case. A mix of nurses with many patients and nurses with only one patient each works best.

One nurse may have more than one patient but each patient has only one primary nurse. This policy, customary in hospice care, is especially important with children because they tend to do better with a minimal degree of change. When children are receiving more than 20 hours a week of private duty care, although they may have several different licensed practical nurses, they still have only one primary nurse. In addition, the private duty nurses always see the same children. Families appreciate the efforts to keep the number of strangers in their home at a minimum.

Clearly this is emotionally difficult work. However, those who do provide the hands-on care of a child who is terminally ill say that there is no greater satisfaction in the clinical profession. They care for the whole family and often are loved as family members long after the child dies.

A nurturing caring atmosphere at the office is necessary as a support system for both in-house clinicians and administrative staff, who deal with the children day after day. As an example, on the day after our annual Memorial Service, when all of us are emotionally drained, we come to work in blue jeans, have lunch together, then spend the afternoon watching comedy videos at the office.

Making the work environment pleasurable is an important part of being effective. Happy, satisfied staff do a better job. Edmarc strives to give its staff equitable salaries, good working conditions, comprehensive benefits, and comfortable working schedules.

WORKING WITH PHYSICIANS

Contrary to the experience of many hospices in the area, Edmarc has outstanding physician support. Although it still struggles with educating the medical community on the need for early referrals, the agency has developed solid working relationships with local physicians. Feedback from these physicians indicates that they are most attracted to the total family care approach, including the sibling and parent support systems, and the sensitivity to the constraints of home-based patient care.

The staff tries to make it easy for the physicians to work with them. For example, the plan of care is written and then sent with orders for approval and signature. Several exceptions are made to the adult hospice rules. It is not required that the physician tell the family that the child is terminal. The patient is accepted on diagnosis if appropriate rather than waiting until the end of life. There are no restrictions on the patients' seeking cure, nor is there a six-month life expectancy rule.

Several prominent local physicians were solicited for quotes to be used in the general brochure. They cited the agency's willingness to take on the toughest cases, its clinical excellence, and its good follow-up. The physicians went on record saying that Edmarc's home care reduced hospital stays. They have frequently been the first point of contact with the families about Edmarc's services, regularly describing its work as compassionate and supportive. The quotes from physicians in our brochure as well as the word-of-mouth reputation are helpful in reinforcing the agency's credibility among other physicians.

The Medical Director is a pediatric oncologist-hematologist who is on staff at the local children's hospital. He is an excellent advocate and spokesperson from within the medical community. He serves in an advisory capacity to the nursing staff and is also a member of the Board of Directors, thus being in a policy-setting position as well as an advisor.

LICENSURE AND CERTIFICATION

Licensure and certification as a home health agency is separate and different from licensure and certification as a hospice. The specific differences are related to the state in which the organization operates. Because Edmarc Hospice for Children is both a home health agency and a hospice, it goes through two regulatory processes.

The home hospice program began by becoming licensed as a home health agency. This turned out to be an important first step because building a reputation as a high caliber home health agency was instrumental in garnering support from the medical community. Licensure also enhances credibility for the general public. The second important step was becoming certified for home health care under Medicare. Although most pediatric patients are not eligible for Medicare coverage, many are under Medicaid or have Blue Cross/Blue Shield coverage, both of which require Medicare certification as a prerequisite for payment in the state of Virginia.

Licensure is through the state Board of Health, and as in any professional health care license, the regulations differ from state to state. In Virginia, a home health license is obtained by writing the appropriate policies and procedures, hiring staff with the appropriate credentials, and allowing the policies and procedures, and medical and personnel records to be examined by surveyors from the Division of Licensure and Certification, Virginia Department of Health.

Edmarc's initial license was only for nursing. As other clinical services were added, such as physical, occupational and speech therapy and medical social services, the agency had to be certified for each service. That process involved hiring or subcontracting with the therapist, writing appropriate policies and procedures, and then notifying the state that the service was to be added. When the paperwork passed, which happened at first submission every time, Edmarc was certified to provide and bill for the service.

Certification for home health under Medicare is very similar to licensure for home health. In fact, in Virginia, the law recently was changed to make Medicare-certified home health agencies exempt from the licensing requirement. The on-site review, or survey, for Medicare certification is also conducted by the Division of Licensure and Certification in Virginia and is the same process as review for licensure. Medicare certification says that the agency meets federal regulations; licensure says that it meets state regulations. However, federal regulations are often more strict than those mandated by the state. In fact, many insurance companies will not establish a provider relationship with a home health agency that is not Medicare certified.

In 1990, Virginia passed a law requiring hospices to be licensed if they use the word "hospice" as a noun in their name. Edmarc Hospice for Children was grandfathered into licensure as soon as it showed that it met all of the standards set by regulation. It is also surveyed annually for continued licensure. Edmarc has opted not to seek Medicare certification as a hospice because these regulations would not accommodate the different admission criteria: that expected remaining life can be longer than six months, that patients are still seeking cure, and that the patients have not necessarily acknowledged terminality.

Since Edmarc does not serve the Medicare population, it does not have to subscribe to many of the Medicare restrictions. However, since Medicare is the primary payor nationally, its regulations are the basis for most state regulations and most third-party payor requirements, and it is wise to keep informed about Medicare legislation.

FUNDING

Edmarc had the luxury of starting with a large private grant that allowed it to offer hospice services throughout the region without regard to the cost of care. The grant served its purpose and was used up within a few years.

However, it has been essential for long-term financial survival to bill for clinical services that are legitimately covered under third-party payment systems (Medicaid, CHAMPUS, Blue Cross/Blue Shield). Third-party payment yields enough income to stretch the agency's capacity to serve even more families. Fifty percent of the annual budget of $500,000 comes from third-party payment.

The operating policy is to give every appropriate patient service whether or not there is any source of payment, but to limit the long-term, expensive care, such as extended private duty nursing, to that which can be reimbursed at least partially.

Edmarc does not expect payment for its services from families for two primary reasons. First, most of the families are young and have very limited financial resources. Any resources they have are usually committed to paying other health-care costs such as hospitalization and physician services. Second, the Board of Directors continues to take the philosophical stance of wanting to provide this service as a ministry and a gift to families.

Some patients' care is individually quite lucrative. For example, there are some cases in which multiple visits are made, which are justifiable and reimbursable, requiring relatively little case management from supervisors. These help us to cover the costs of the cases where there are many visits that are not reimbursable. The goal of third-party payors often does not fit well with the goal of pediatric hospice. Third-party payors want to pay for improvement and for rehabilitation aimed at achieving self-sufficiency so that the patient will need less care. Clearly, it is hard to justify continued improvement with children who are progressively declining. Therefore, the staff tries to cite improvements in specific modalities: in physical therapy that could mean a percentage improvement in movement in one arm; in skilled nursing that could mean a decrease in the number of infections or a decrease in hospital days. Sometimes, it is necessary to just take the loss. It is not realistic to assume that pediatric hospice will be financially self-sufficient.

Philanthropic dollars are needed to support a great deal of unpaid care and many nonbillable services such as volunteer coordination, community education, bereavement care, and family support services. Fifty percent of Edmarc's budget comes from philanthropy of one sort or another. Although it is easier to raise money to care for sick children than for many other causes, it took a long time to build a donor base. Potential donors needed to be aware of the available services and the need for funds before they could give. The agency now has a very high percentage of repeat donors. Fifteen percent of the budget comes from individual and group donations. Many gifts are received in memory of the children who have been served or in memory of a family member or friend. An annual direct mail solicitation of all former donors is done every Christmas and raises a substantial amount of money.

Ten percent of the budget comes from United Way; another 20 percent comes from grants and foundations. Grants are an especially good vehicle both for getting new programs started and for capital items, such as computers or medical equipment. Foundations, especially those that are directed to provide services for a particular community, are a good source for repeat support.

The agency's church affiliation provides contact with people who are prone to giving to church-related causes. Churches and synagogues, in general, are a good source of funds, volunteers, and resources such as space for meetings.

Once Edmarc experienced a solid, predictable increase in donations and grants such that it was in the black for a reasonable period of time, it used funds to add new staff, representing new programs. A volunteer program, a bereavement program, and social work services would have started much sooner if more money had been available. However, the improved services actually helped to bring in more money because the agency was more marketable to potential donors.

The Board of Directors must understand that one of its primary functions is to raise money to further the agency's mission. Edmarc staff historically has expended paid time raising money that could have been raised through board efforts.

Volunteers have been a valuable resource for raising money through fund-raising events, such as regular flea markets, cookbook sales, and a Sponsor-A-Family program. These efforts yield 5% of our budget.

COLLEGIAL RELATIONS

Edmarc's liberal admission criteria, willingness to make reasonable exceptions to any rule, efforts to be holistic in service, and striving for clinical excellence helped it to build a reputation as a fair and caring agency. This public recognition enabled Edmarc to build both physician and financial support.

The staff found it very helpful to be involved with their other hospice colleagues to share new ideas and obtain answers to problems within the organization. Without ongoing contact with adult hospice providers, staff could easily lose touch with recent trends in hospice care.

Since Edmarc operates under the aegis of a home health agency, it benefits from participation in the local home care association. Trusted home care colleagues share information on current salary and charge structures, from which the agency can base its operating decisions. It is kept abreast of rapidly changing regulations, shares resources for continuing education and staff development, and learns from each other.

MARKETING AND PUBLIC RELATIONS

Most of our marketing efforts are in one of two forms: speaking engagements and a newsletter. Nothing is more effective as a marketing tool than the one-to-one telling of our story. Invitations are actively solicited to speak to any group size. Edmarc has a ten-minute video, produced with grant money, which is usually accompanied by a ten- to fifteen-minute presentation by a staff member. Groups regularly respond with a donation of money or volunteers. The newsletter is produced five times a year, bimonthly and one for the summer months. This newsletter is sent to all donors and any interested groups and individuals who we want to be kept informed about program developments. All donations are published in the newsletter and it is believed that the listing helps to produce more donations.

CONCLUSION

Although pediatric hospice care is terribly sad, it is not always depressing because it is filled with hope. It seems to bring out the very best in people—nurses who go way beyond the call of duty; parents who love and care for their children with more devotion and selflessness than one could imagine possible. When a beloved family member is dying, time takes on a different quality. Every moment becomes a memory. The impact of hospice work lasts more than a lifetime—it lasts through the lifetimes of every family member. When staff can have a positive impact on the quality of life of a dying child and thereby have a positive impact on that family's experience of grief, they have given the gift of greater peace during bereavement. Conversely, it is a gift to be involved with these families, if only to offer companionship. The love and the willingness to connect are the sources of real healing.

A Home Care Program

IDA MARTINSON

Home care for dying children could be an option for most families throughout the United States. Home Care for the Child with Cancer, a nursing research study funded by the National Cancer Institute and conducted from 1976 to 1978, demonstrated the feasibility and the desirability of home care for dying children. Numerous publications are available describing this study and other aspects of providing care to the terminally ill child.[1-12] From 1978 to 1980, the program was continued through ongoing hospital agencies and this section will deal with the results from that phase which previously has not been reported. This section will also include an update of the present situation in the same geographical area, the use of varieties of the model elsewhere, and recommendations.

BACKGROUND

As late as the mid-1970s, children were admitted to the hospital when their dying was no longer preventable. In the Home Care for the Child with Cancer Project, physicians, however, were willing to consider home care as an alternative to the hospital when death was inevitable. Nurses were recruited to have the responsibility of 24-hour on-call and be supportive to the families who desired to meet their child's wish to be at home at the end of life. Thus a new model of care was developed.

A second goal of the Home Care for the Child with Cancer Project was to assist existing facilities in taking over pediatric hospice/home care, based on the model for hospice/home care that was developed in 1976–78. During 1978–80, the transferring of the direct home care services from the Project to existing community facilities took place.

Institutional Involvement

Three institutions with a sizable pediatric oncology population indicated an interest in collaborating with the Project and were chosen as the major institutions for involvement during the Project's last two years (1978–80). The three institutions were the University of Minnesota, Minneapolis Children's Health Center, and the St. Louis Park Medical Clinic.

The University of Minnesota is a large teaching and referral center located on the Minneapolis campus of the university. At that time, 40% of the patients were from the Twin Cities metropolitan area, 38% from outlying counties in Minnesota, and 22% were from out of state. The hospital has six pediatric wards and one neonatal intensive care unit; children with cancer are admitted to all these areas depending on age and condition. The University of Minnesota Hospitals initiated a Home Health Services Department in September 1974. In July 1978, this department also assumed the provision for 24-hour direct nursing care for children dying at home in the Twin Cities metropolitan area from the Home Care for the Child with Cancer Project. In addition, the home care staff also provided indirect coordination and consultation to nurses in public health nursing agencies caring for children referred to them by the University of Minnesota Hospitals.

Minneapolis Children's Health Center is a 107-bed private pediatric hospital in Minneapolis that serves children aged 0 to 21 years. This hospital's home care program was instituted in July 1978. It is coordinated by a master's-prepared nurse who was hired in June 1978 to develop and direct the program. This program began with assuming the pediatric hospice/home care responsibilities of the Home Care for the Child with Cancer Project.

St. Louis Park Medical Center is a large, multispecialty outpatient clinic founded in 1951. Approximately 110 pediatric hematology-oncology patients receive clinic services annually. In May 1978, a home care program was instituted as the first phase of the Home Care for the Child with Cancer Project concluded. The nurse coordinator and the two pediatric-oncologists followed their patients from referral through death. The children who earlier were referred to the Home Care for the Child with Cancer Project were now managed by their own institutions.

During the last eighteen months of the Home Care for the Child with Cancer Project, 37 children were referred to the institutions' own home care programs. The Project staff continued with data collection with these families. Twenty-three children died, of which 5 families refused to participate in the data collection aspects of the project. Of these 18 children, 11

(61%) were males and 7 (39%) were females, this sex ratio (7/11 or .64) is similar to the first study (21/37 or .57). At death, the age of the children ranged from 2 through 13 years; the mean age was 6.6 years. Of the families included, 44% resided in the Twin Cities metropolitan area, 39% resided in other areas throughout Minnesota, and 17% resided in neighboring states. The rural-urban mix was very similar to the first study as reported. All the parents were Caucasian and there were no major differences in the socioeconomic status, religious preferences, or educational level from the first study.

Children Characteristics

The children had a wide range of diagnoses with leukemia being the most common. All of the children were alert and oriented at the onset of home care, but at some point during the process of home care, 72% of the children were comatose or semicomatose. Physical symptoms noted during home care included difficulties in breathing, drinking, and eating by two-thirds of the children. Vomiting occurred in about three-fourths of the cases and ten of the children had some bleeding. No decubitus ulcers were noted in any of the children.

Home Care Features

The duration of home care services received by the families ranged from 2 to 445 days. More than half (56%) of the children received home care for two weeks or less while two children were in the program for more than three months, one for 139 days and the other for 445 days. The mean number of days of home care was 53.5 days and the median was 14 days.

As reported by Moldow and colleagues,[8] the cost of home care for dying children was compared with hospital costs. Depending on the comparison groups used, the costs for hospital care are about 22 to 207% more than home care. Variation in comparisons depends on whether the home care is purely an alternative to inpatient hospitalization or representative of a larger concept of care that includes added services at times when the child would not necessarily be hospitalized.

As in the earlier study, families' needs for nursing assistance varied widely. Some families wanted to remain independent and felt capable of managing the child by themselves; in other instances, the nurse was very involved with the family. The average family received 12.1 home visits with a total average time of 16.2 hours. However, the number of visits per family ranged from 1 to 27 and the total time ranged from 50 minutes to 83 hours. Parents reported the 24-hour availability of the nurse as an extremely important facet of home care and that the ready accessibility of the nurse by telephone was very comforting.

The home care nurses ranged in age from 21 to 64 years with a mean age of 35.7 years. The majority of the nurses held either a bachelor's degree or a diploma in nursing. Total years of nursing experience ranged from 2.5 years to 34 years with a mean of 10.6 years. Years of public health nursing experience ranged from 0 to 28 years, with a mean of 3 years. Forty-one percent of the nurses had pediatric experience. All families received educational services from their physicians, while 78% received assessment services and 83% received emotional and supportive care. As in the earlier study, the role of other health professionals was minimal. One family received 29 visits from a home health aide, 1 from an occupational therapist, and 1 from a physical therapist. In addition, two families used educational tutors for their children and five families received visits from clergy during the home care period. While social workers were involved with the families during the child's stay in the hospital, on returning to their homes in the rural area, these relationships did not continue until after the death of the child.

Pain and Symptom Control

Pain control was of primary importance. All children received pain medications; 56% received a narcotic analgesic, 33% received a combination of narcotic analgesic and antianxiety medication, and 11% received a non-narcotic analgesic. Some of the school-age children were afraid of becoming addicted or immune to the pain medications; however, the children did agree to take the prescribed pain medications after discussing their fears with the home care nurse.

Other medications were used for symptom control and comfort in addition to pain control. The number of medications received by children while they were at home ranged from 0 to 12; the mean number of medications was 4.9 and the median was 3.5. The variety of equipment and supplies reflects the variation in the condition of the children receiving home care and the creativity of both home care nurses and families in meeting the needs of these children.

Comparison Group Children

All families whose child was under the care of a physician at these institutions and who died in the hospital from cancer, whether or not treatment had been stopped, became the basis for a comparison group. Each child's physician was contacted to determine whether the child was or was not receiving cure-oriented treatment at the time of death and if the family had been offered home care services. Permission to contact the family was also obtained from the physician. For each case, information was abstracted from patient records. In addition, each family was contacted and requested to participate in the study. During this phase, 51 children who were treated at the three cooperating institutions died. Four were judged as inappropriate for home care and were excluded for the following reasons: one child died immediately after surgery, another was in the hospital for only one day receiving only diagnostic services, a third child had an unexpected hospital admission with loss of consciousness and died within 24 hours of admission, and the fourth family had returned their child for a final course of chemotherapy. Of the remaining 47 children who could have received home care services, 57% participated in home care and 53% did not participate. Of the 25 children who did not participate in home care, 20 were receiving active cure-oriented treatment at the time of death.

Table A.1 shows that 3 of the 5 comparison group children who were not receiving curative treatment were offered home care. For one of these families home care was arranged, but the child died before being discharged from the hospital. Another family was offered home care but preferred to care for their child at home without formal involvement in the home care project. A third family was offered home care but chose to keep the child in the hospital because the mother felt that only the hospital could provide

Table A.1   Treatment Groups

		Number of Families
Children not receiving curative treatment		
Offered, accepted, not enough time to set up home care		1
Offered home care, refused		2
Not offered home care		2
	Subtotal	5
Children receiving curative treatment		
Offered, accepted, not enough time to set up home care		2
Offered home care, refused, wanted more treatment		1
Physician thought home care not appropriate		1
Not offered home care because death was not expected		16
	Subtotal	20

the supportive care that her child needed for comfort and because she did not want the child's siblings to observe what she felt would be a difficult death.

Table A.1 also shows that some of the children who were receiving curative treatment were also offered home care. Two of these families accepted home care but in each case the child died before home care services could be arranged. The one family who refused home care felt they wanted the support of the hospital through the time of death and chose to try another course of chemotherapy.

Interviews with these parents provide some insight as to why parents decided not to choose home care. In one case, the mother said that she thought of taking her child home but was discouraged by the child's need for a respirator and intravenous feedings, and by the child's many seizures the last two days of life. Another mother said that she would have chosen home care because other relatives had died at home, but when the child was placed on a respirator she decided not to pursue home care. Another mother who took her child home returned to the hospital when the child developed severe pain. The mother's decision was also influenced by her wish for the child to receive pain medications and intravenous fluids so that she would not feel her child was starving to death. One father said there "just wasn't time . . . for home care" and "in this situation the child would have to be in the hospital." Another family said they thought their child would survive until two days before death, were hoping for a bone marrow transplant, and would never have considered going home. Another mother wanted to take her child home but felt the physical complications the child developed would have been "too much" for the siblings.

STUDY CONCLUSIONS

The most obvious conclusion of this research is that home care for children dying of cancer is feasible when coordinated through the research nursing staff as well as by the home care programs in health-care institutions. Home care can be provided and that care can become a regular part of the community health-care system. The provision of care to children with a variety of cancer diagnoses and widely varying physical conditions, of a wide range of ages and living in families of diverse socioeconomic, occupational, and educational backgrounds leads to the conclusion that there are no reasons why home care should be ruled out a priori on the basis of these factors.

The fact that nurses were recruited for home care without great difficulty and that almost all home care nurses were able to complete the cases they began strongly suggests that home care is feasible from the nurse's perspective. That about two-thirds of the home care nurses would provide this care again and that three-fourths would recommend their agency provide this type of care also suggest that home care is viewed as desirable by these nurses both for themselves and the agencies for which they work.

Similarly, the variety of educational and occupational backgrounds represented among the nurses who provided home care supports the conclusion that nurses can provide home care to children dying of cancer. While nurses can be effective in the provision of home care while employed in another job, there is evidence that the home care nurse must be available on a 24-hour basis. Data from some cases where the child was readmitted to the hospital suggest that those readmissions may be related to the occurrence of physical problems in the child which could not be controlled by parents and inability of the home care nurse to respond in time to the parents' calls for help.

ROLE OF PARENTS, NURSES, AND PHYSICIANS

Parents

The study has demonstrated that parents can provide the majority of care for children who are dying of cancer, even when these children exhibit a wide variety of very serious problems. Most certainly the nurse's ability to teach parents how to care for their child and to provide emotional support, along with the consultation of the physician, are key elements in the provision of home care.

Nurses

Home care nurses must be able to develop solutions to problems that they may well not have dealt with before. This means they must be both flexible and creative. There is ample evidence of very wide variability in the quantitative aspects of the care provided and of the individual approach each family/nurse/physician took to the care of the child they were concerned with. The model of care that has evolved in this project is purposefully broad so as to encourage the type of individualization that occurred. It is clear that the nurses who undertook the care in that model were able to maximize that flexibility.

Physicians

The physician's role in this model represents a departure for most physicians. Pediatric oncologists remained very much involved with local pediatricians, in some instances, assisting in the care of the child at home. Because the physician seldom visited the child at home and because clinic-office visits were infrequent, physicians relied heavily on the observation, interpretation, and judgments of both nurses and parents. Particularly in the area of medications, physicians had to depend on the home care nurse for judgments and/or recommendations in dosages and on the nurse and family for administration.

CRITICAL NOTES

Information in this study shows that the control of pain and other symptoms is of primary importance in the provision of home care. However, there are no particular symptoms or conditions that always lead parents to rehospitalize their children. Thus, while some parents preferred for their child to return to the hospital for problems such as bleeding or abscesses, other parents chose to deal with those problems at home. While a considerable amount of medical technology was brought to bear in many of the home care cases, almost all parents tried to maintain the atmosphere and identity of the home. Thus few hospital beds and other hospital furnishings were used. Moreover, in many cases the locus of home care was not the child's bedroom but the living room or family room of the home; a place where the dying child could participate more easily in the affairs of the family.

Almost one out of every five children who entered home care died in the hospital. There were no differences between children who died at home and those who died in the hospital. Children who died in the hospital were neither more or less severely affected by their disease than children who died at home. There were relationships between death at home and both the number of medications used and the rate of home visits by the nurse. Also where children died at home, home care nurses made more telephone calls, and more supplies and equipment were used. Children who received more intensive home care were more likely to die at home.

The research also clearly demonstrated that home care for children dying from cancer is feasible from a cost standpoint. Whether the cost of home care is considered on an average daily basis or on an average total basis, that cost is consistently and considerably less than the cost of comparable care provided in the hospital.

Parents' Satisfaction with Home Care

While parents were generally satisfied with the home care their children received, there were some differences in this area between parents of children who died at home and parents of children who died in the hospital. Twelve months after the child's death only three parents expressed any degree of dissatisfaction with the nursing services provided. However, because these three parents (representing two families) were parents of children who died in the hospital, there is some concern that the dissatisfaction with nursing care was related to the decision to rehospitalize the child. Also, when asked (12 months after the child's death) whether they would choose home care again, 97% of parents whose child died at home but only 38% of those whose child died in the hospital said they definitely would choose home care again. But when this question was repeated 24 months after the child's death, 96% of all parents said they would choose home care again. Again, though, those few parents expressing uncertainty were parents of a child who died in the hospital. Furthermore, parents of children who died in the hospital were more likely than parents of children who died at home to say they would change their child's treatment if they had it to do over again and also more likely to report that they would change some aspects of the child's time at home before death. Finally, when asked to identify specific events that stood out in memory of their child's last days at home, parents of children who died at home were more likely than parents of children who died in the hospital to identify a positive aspect of that time.

Thus, in contrast to parents of children who died at home, parents of children who died in the hospital are more likely to recall negative events of home care and less likely to recall positive events. These parents are also more likely to say they would have treated their child's cancer differently and more likely to say they would change something about the home care their child received. It would appear, then, that parents of children who died at home have fewer negative and more positive feelings about their child's home care than do parents of children who died in the hospital. While it is not possible to say whether these feelings either derive from or lead to the decision to rehospitalize the dying child, it is clear that the parents of children who died at home do not hold negative feelings toward their decision to keep their child at home.

Parent's Identification of Positive Aspects

Parents' responses to the request to identify positive aspects of home care show that the care met many different needs in the families involved. In general, the comments regarding positive aspects for dying children seem to indicate that parents felt their children wanted to be at home and that once the child got home and was no longer separated from the family, the child felt better emotionally (happier, more secure, more relaxed), and also better physically. The comments also suggest that parents believed their children could live more normally at home and could achieve more control over their lives by asking for and accepting personal care and involvement in family activities when they wanted it. When commenting on benefits for themselves, parents identified how disruptive the child's illness had been to the family and how home care helped to change that. Parents also mentioned that home care allowed them to be able to care for their own child and to be nearby 24 hours a day. In addition, parents felt they had more control at home saying that "home care afforded us full control of the situation" and "home care was a feeling of being in full control, providing a normal environment for our family." The quality of nursing services and the availability of the nurse were two positive aspects mentioned most often by parents in regard to actual home care services received.

Parents Identification of Negative Aspects

Home care parents also expressed some negative comments. In general, though, parents identified fewer negative aspects than they did positive aspects and the negative aspects which were identified were less likely than the positive aspects to be made by more than one or two parents. Most of the negative comments generally reflect the stress parents felt as a result of the child's care, illness, and death. Five parents reported that home care was "exhausting," four parents said that it was difficult to keep well-meaning visitors away, and three parents mentioned the need for more follow-up and the management of medication.

Parental Concerns Regarding Death Itself

A major concern of many home care parents (and of others familiar with this model of care) has been the actual death of the child at home. In particular, there has been concern that parents would have difficulty confronting the medical and physiological aspects of their child's death at home and, as a consequence, would require the presence of home care nurses and other professionals at the time of death. On the other hand, a primary benefit anticipated for home care was that it would allow the parents to gather family and friends around them for support at the time of the child's death, a situation that would not always be possible in a hospital. Because of these concerns, parents were asked (during the interview one month after the child's death) to relate who was present (i.e., in the child's room or just outside in an adjacent room or hallway) at the time their child died. Both parents and other relatives were more likely to be with the child at the time of death if that death took place at home rather than in the hospital. Furthermore, nurses were present at one-third of the deaths that occurred at home and only three-fourths of the deaths that occurred in the hospital. It is apparent that families do not necessarily require the presence of the home care nurse at the time of death. Moreover, because several families purposefully waited until after the child's death to call the nurse, it may well be that some families prefer to manage the child's death without the nurse's assistance.

Responses of Nurses to Home Care

The major index of feasibility in terms of home care nurses concerned whether nurses could be found to provide home care services and whether they would complete their home care assignment, once they had begun. At the outset of the Project, coordinators had some difficulty finding home care nurses, particularly when the family lived in a community which was remote from the Twin Cities or in which provision of home care for dying children had not been tried. However, there were no instances in either of the studies where a referral was refused because a home care nurse could not be found. Moreover, in the two cases where the original home care nurse could not complete her home care assignment, another nurse was recruited without difficulty. From the standpoint of finding nurses willing to provide services to a number of families distributed over a large geographical area, then, home care appears quite feasible. Again, that about two-thirds of the home care nurses would provide this care again and that three-fourths would recommend their agency provide this type of care also suggest that home care is viewed as desirable by these nurses both for themselves and the agencies for which they work.

The nurse's need for and use of emotional support was a major concern in this study. In both studies, nurses identified their own family and friends as the group most supportive. Many nurses identified their husband as their primary source of support and the nurse's parents, particularly a mother, were often referred to as sources of support who contributed to "renewed feelings of energy." Such support was highly valued. Conversely, other nurses voiced their disappointment in the failure to develop family support systems. The majority of nurses spoke of support from nursing colleagues (fellow hospital and public health agency staff, nursing supervisors, back-up nurses, nursing instructors, and nursing in-service staff). These nurses frequently noted they could speak to colleagues freely, in a way that was not possible with others. Staff support helped them resolve some of their feelings regarding the death of specific children.

Included among the emotional support mechanisms identified by the nurses was the support provided by the research project coordinators and home care coordinators. Nurses commented on the concern, interest, and availability of the research nursing coordinators or the institutional home care coordinators. They also referred specifically to the reassurance, moral support, shared feelings, and answers to questions provided by these staff members. The telephone availability of home care coordinators was also considered particularly helpful to home care nurses. In addition, other health-care professionals contributed emotional, physical, and technical support to the home care nurses.

It is apparent then that nurses need emotional support during the provision of home care and that they develop a variety of mechanisms for obtaining that support.

Responses of Physicians to Home Care

Because physicians are one of the keys to the success of home care in that they refer children to that care, physicians involved in the project were surveyed to determine their attitudes. Of the 37 physicians involved in both phases of the project, 29 (78%) agreed to be interviewed. All responded that they would use home care services again. No differences in responses were found according to the physician's form of medical practice or specialty. Physicians sharing these positive feelings saw the use of home care as an integral part of their medical practice. Almost all physicians felt that home care provided psychological advantages to the family. Physicians also viewed the assessment of needs in the home situation as a major advantage of home care. Because many of the needs are not apparent in the hospital or office setting, it is important for the nurse to make these observations in the home. Physicians said they were better able to treat the family by knowing of these needs.

A number of physicians emphasized that communication between the physician and home care nurse is an extremely important aspect of the care. Some physicians were concerned that the home care nurse might assume too much responsibility and fail to report important changes to the physician. It was stressed that findings need to be related to the physician, particularly in regard to side effects of medication. Differing philosophies (between nurses and physicians) in this area were seen as a potential source of confusion and anxiety for families. Within this area, legal aspects of home care were discussed by only a few. However, the consensus of opinion among the physicians interviewed was that close contact among the physician, family, and nurse would assure the absence of any legal questions.

Both through their referrals to this program and by participating in home care and responding to the interviews, physicians have demonstrated the feasibility of home care for dying children. Satisfaction with home care and the pattern of repeated referrals from physicians in the community leave little doubt that home care is feasible from the physician's perspective. The repeated referrals, the positive responses, and the general level of support among physicians in the community certainly suggest that many regard home care for dying children as not only feasible but also desirable for a sizable portion of families with dying children.

Institutionalization of Home Care

Several measures of feasibility relate to the institutionalization of the home care model. Staff and administration support at all three institutions has been excellent, and physicians, nurses, clergy, and others have continued to refer cases to home care at approximately the same rate. There were no apparent differences in the home care services provided by nurses, physicians, or others. While each institution altered the home care model developed earlier to accommodate the uniqueness of each institution and patient population, essentially similar home care was provided. A major concern of the research staff and medical community was whether this type of home care service would be covered by existing health insurance plans. However, in all but one family, existing health care plans paid a large portion or all of the cost.

These data, combined with the development of similar programs in Seattle, Los Angeles, and Milwaukee, and with survey results showing the feasibility of most elements of the model in county nursing agencies, show that pediatric hospice/home care can now be provided by health-care institutions in the community.

Situation Update with the Three Institutions

St. Louis Park Medical Center merged with Children's Hospital into a joint program. The Children's Hospital in Minneapolis has the largest home care services. With a staff of 94 or the equivalent to 60 full-time staff they make 2046 home visits per month. In this program approximately 15 children die a year and 60 to 70% die at home with the support from the nursing team. While oncology patients are still the most common for hospice care, they also care for children with inoperable heart or cardiac myopathy as well as degenerative neuromuscular diseases. The director is the same director, Becky Bedore, who began the program. The University of Minnesota home care department reports that in 1992 there were 10 children involved in hospice/home care. Their team serves families within a thirty-minute radius of the university and the special houses such as Ronald McDonald for children with cancer or the special house for liver and kidney patients. They also work with families who have a terminally ill child in other public health agencies throughout the area.

PITFALLS IN PEDIATRIC HOSPICE HOME CARE

Major pitfalls in the establishment of pediatric hospice/home care is the tendency for too elaborate teams to be established for the number of children served. Consultations need to be established first with the links to the expertise needed in the care of pediatric children. While nurses are willing to consult with physicians, clergy, social workers, and other health care professionals, too often the links to nurse consultants have not been developed.

RECOMMENDATIONS

The research led to a number of recommendations, which are reported below. Most of these recommendations flow directly from the findings and conclusions already discussed. Others, though, derive from more general knowledge and sensitivities that the researchers have received from the conduct of this project.

Primary among the recommendations is that home care for children dying of cancer be made available as an alternative for families desiring it. This study has shown that home care can be provided to children in a large geographic area through the development of one or a few programs. Such care should become an alternative offered by major cancer treatment centers and other institutions in the community such as adult hospices or the public health nursing agencies.

Other recommendations include the following:

- A program of education and support for the families and friends of home care nurses should be developed at least on a pilot basis. Although there are a number of innovative programs that provide support for human services staff dealing with life-threatening or highly stressful diseases, no facilities have been identified that offer a systematic educational or emotionally supportive program to the family members and friends that support these staff.
- The condition of the nurse's home/family situation should be considered in choosing nurses to provide home care. This recommendation reflects the finding that the support given by the nurse's family is often a key to her coping with the stress of home care.
- Because one-third of the children who entered home care died within the first two weeks, the home care nurse should make an initial visit within the first 24 hours of home care.

- Particularly in cases where home care extended over several weeks, home care nurses should offer to provide "respite care" for parents. This might include staying with the dying child while the parents go out for an evening or staying awake with the child while the parents sleep.

- If parents choose to keep their dying child in the hospital (or to readmit the child to the hospital from home care), the hospital should make provision for continued involvement of the parents in the child's care.

- Hospital nursing staff and physicians should maintain contact with home care families after they leave the hospital and especially after the child's death.

- A pilot program should be undertaken to provide follow-up with parents for an extended period (2 years and beyond). This follow-up should be conducted by trained parent advocates or counselors. Many parents reported having benefited from such interviews conducted as part of this project.

- Because children in home care may suddenly develop needs for pain medications, home care nurses should obtain orders for such medication on admission to home care and should have available the necessary supplies, etc. to administer the medication.

- At least some aspects of the home care model should begin earlier in the disease than at the point of deciding to cease curative treatment. Information from this study (particularly in regard to the stress parents feel from the time of the child's diagnosis through his/her death) suggest the benefit of beginning the process of home care at the time of diagnosis.

- Education should be provided to parents regarding the physiological processes of death. In particular, parents need to know what might happen to their child just before death and what death will "look" like.

- Because many of the problems encountered in home care of dying children do not have routine solutions, home care programs should provide training in creative problem solving for nurses. Also, information on how various problems have been solved should be recorded and communicated among nurses by coordinators and the use of journals, notebooks, and case presentations.

- Further examination of parents' grieving processes should be undertaken with a long-term perspective recognizing that, in this study, many parents were grieving 24 months after the child's death.

- Because parent support groups were used by most of the parents in this study who felt they needed support, such groups should be more widely developed and made available to parents of dying and deceased children.

- Because this study could identify no particular "family type" which was either "not appropriate" or "most appropriate" for home care, health professionals should use criteria other than family characteristics in deciding who should be referred to home care.
- Similarly, because little difference was found in the performance of nurses on the basis of their education or experience, other factors should be considered in choosing home care nurses. The coordinator would need to have pediatric preparation and experience to be able to advise the home care nurses of special needs based on the child's developmental level.
- The home care model could be extended to include services to children with chronic and other end-stage diseases.
- Because it may be that "routinizing" home care leads to lower satisfaction of parents, home care programs should consider using only nurses who are especially interested in and committed to home care for dying children.
- Special attention should be devoted to selection and preparation of the home care coordinator. Because this person selects and trains the nurses, assigns them to cases, monitors performance, and is involved to some extent with every case in his/her agency, the home care coordinator is both essential to the program and subject to a great deal of stress.
- Home care programs should consider the provision of homemaker assistance to families involved in home care. Many of the families in this project benefited from help in areas such as washing dishes, house cleaning, and meal preparation.

NOTES

1. Gronseth E, Martinson IM (1981). Support system of health professionals as observed in the project of home care for the child with cancer. Death Education 5(1):37–50.

2. Martinson IM, Henry WF (1980). Some possible societal consequences of changing the way in which we care for dying children. Hastings Center Report 10: 5–8.

3. Martinson, IM, Nixon, S, Geis, D, YaDeau, R, Nesbit, M, Kersey, J (1982). Nursing care in childhood cancer: Methadone. American Journal of Nursing, March:432–435.

4. Martinson IM, Nesbit M, Kersey J (1985). Physician's role in home care for children with cancer. Death Studies 9:283–293.

5. Martinson IM, Davies EB, McClowry SG (1987). The long-term effects of sibling death on self-concept. Journal of Pediatric Nursing 2:227–235.

6. Martinson IM, Moldow DG, Armstrong GA, Henry WF, Kersey J, Nesbit M

(1986). Home care for children dying with cancer. Research in Nursing and Health 2:11–16.

7. McClowry SG, Davies EB, May KA, Kulenkamp EJ, Martinson IM (1987). The empty space phenomenon: The process of grief in the bereaved family. Death Studies 11:361–374.

8. Moldow DG, Armstrong GD, Henry WF, Martinson IM (1982). The cost of home care for dying children. Medical Care 20:1114–1160.

9. Moldow DG, Martinson IM (1980). From research to reality: Home care for the dying child. MCN: The American Journal of Maternal Child Nursing 51: 1159–1160, 1162, 1166.

10. Martinson IM, Campos RG (1991). Adolescent bereavement: Long term responses to a sibling's death from cancer. Journal of Adolescent Research 6:54–69.

11. Martinson IM, Birenbaum L, Martin B, Lauer M, Ing B (1991). Hospice/ Home Care: A Nurses' Manual for Management for Children. Children's Hospice International, Alexandria, VA.

12. Moldow DG, Martinson IM (1991). Parents' Manual for Seriously Ill Children at Home. Children's Hospice International, Alexandria, VA.

Palliative Care in an Inpatient Hospital Setting

NEIL LOMBARDI

St. Mary's Free Hospital for Children was founded in 1870 as the first Children's Hospital in New York. In 1985, St. Mary's dedicated the first inpatient pediatric Palliative Care Unit in the United States. This ten bed unit is part of a ninety-five bed pediatric skilled nursing facility — St. Mary's Hospital for Children in Bayside, New York — devoted primarily to rehabilitation of infants and children with chronic disorders. It is also part of a larger Palliative Care Program that provides comprehensive home care and day care services to terminally ill children and their families. (The terms *palliative care program* and *hospice* are used here interchangeably, although they may have different connotations and/or regulatory implications in various states.) This section of the appendix will describe our experience with the inpatient unit, its development, growth, and function, and provide the reader with a perspective on its programs and implications.[1]

HISTORICAL BACKGROUND

Before describing our experience with inpatient palliative care at St. Mary's Hospital for Children, it is important that I provide the reader with a perspective on how I became involved in this field. When I first entered pediatric residency training, the subject of death in childhood was not a topic of discussion. It was generally considered that the objective of all our ministrations was the survival of the child, no matter how ill, at all costs. Thus the thought that a child might die while in our care was suppressed until the inevitable occurred. We were not prepared for it nor were we capable of preparing the child or the family for what could be predicted in many instances to be inevitable. As the time drew near and the child became aware of the terminal nature of his or her condition, the denial on the part of the treating staff became more and more firm. Frequently, this denial led to an avoidance of the child and the family in order to reduce the chances of having to discuss the nearing demise. We would round quickly past the child's room, going in only to make specific observations or do procedures, and little or no conversation ensued. There was an acknowledged lack of personal emotional resources, and specifically a lack of knowledge as to how and when to discuss the possibility with either the family or the child that the child might die. Sometimes the child asked, but the parents almost never did. And when the child asked, the response was usually in the form of a terse reassurance, thus compounding the conspiracy of silence. Inevitably a painful wall was built between the child, the family, and the caretakers; a wall of abandonment based on an overwhelming need to deny the inevitable.

This frustration, combined with a sense of the need to identify terminally ill children and assist them, their families, and caregivers to acknowledge and cope with the pain of death in childhood, was the impetus that led to the development of the Palliative Care Program at St. Mary's Hospital for Children. And so, when confronted with the opportunity of participating in the development of this program when I began to consult for St. Mary's Hospital for Children, I embraced the idea with a great deal of enthusiasm, having in mind those vivid memories of my training years and the need to do something different and hopefully more caring and effective for children with terminal illnesses. (The details of how the program was developed will be discussed later under "Process of Development" and "Defining a Site.")

It is very important to be aware of the historical context in which these attitudes toward death in children developed. Just sixty years ago, William Carlos Williams, a physician and poet, described what it was like to practice medicine in the preantibiotic, preimmunization era.[2] Death in children was frequent from common diseases such as diphtheria or bacterial meningitis. During the next fifty years, the development of antibiotics, immunizations, chemotherapeutic agents, radiation, and surgical techniques would arrive that would give the pediatrician the sense that all disease in childhood was either preventable or curable. It was during this period of time that pediatricians were prone to deny the possibility of death or dying in children. However, as the focus turned to the nature of chronic illness, physicians were again confronted with the reality that despite the many wonderful medical advances, there were still many children dying, often after long bouts with chronic illnesses. We had not found "cures" for many progressive, metabolic, and degenerative disorders of the central nervous system.

There were still many childhood tumors that responded poorly to radiation and chemotherapy. Children were being born with lethal congenital malformations that were not amenable to surgery, or chromosomal abnormalities or neuromuscular disorders that led to their inevitable death within a year or so of birth or, as with other disorders, not until adolescence or even young adulthood.

In the past ten years, we have been confronted with a new disease AIDS, which affects not only the child, but also the mother who is the source of the virus to her infant. The full impact of this epidemic has not yet been felt, but it presents us with the peculiar challenge of caring for the dying child and dying mother at the same time.

It is in this context that there has been the renewal of interest in the management of chronic illness and terminal illness in childhood, and it is in this context that planning began for the development of a pediatric palliative care program at St. Mary's. It must be emphasized, however, there is still a great deal of variation on the part of pediatricians and pediatric subspecialists in their attitude toward the approach to a child with a terminal illness. There is still a great deal of resistance of many to come to grips with the inevitability of death under many circumstances, and there are still those who are very uncomfortable at identifying a point where medical intervention is no longer useful or appropriate.[3,4] In addition, it must be pointed out that advances in the treatment of children with chronic illnesses are continuing to evolve, and certain diseases (especially childhood malignancies) have seen remarkable increases in long-term survival rates, making the definition and identification of that point more and more difficult.

EVALUATION OF APPROPRIATENESS FOR INPATIENT CARE

The inpatient unit of our comprehensive Palliative Care Program at St. Mary's Hospital for Children consists of a ten-bed inpatient skilled nursing unit. Selection of patients appropriate for this unit is a complex task involving prediction of life expectancy, evaluation of patient and family needs, attitudes, and expectations as well as determination of the acuity of the illness and symptomatic involvement of the child.

The task of predicting life expectancy of a child with a terminal diagnosis has proved much more elusive than originally thought. As initially conceived, the limited bed space would be reserved for those families desirous of inpatient treatment whose children had a life expectancy of six months or less. Although pediatric texts and literature describe the life expectancy of certain congenital malformations (e.g., anencephaly or hydranenceph-aly) as being days to weeks,[5-7] we have had the experience of caring for a number of children with such abnormalities for months and even years! As we gain experience with various illnesses thought to be lethal in the short run, we have become less and less sure about our predictions of life expectancy. Frequently, however, parents come to us having been given quite definitive statements about the potential duration of survival with certain conditions. In view of the discrepancy between what is disseminated in the literature and our personal experiences, we are often in a position of supporting the ambivalent feelings of the families.

Many feel that involvement with "hospice" or "palliative care" means the abandonment of "hope." Our experiences led us to the conclusion that seeking hospice services in no way excludes the possibility of more pro-longed survival. It is not necessary, or even practical, to consider the decision to seek palliative care as mutually exclusive of ongoing treatment, and indeed the values involved suggest a more reasonable "dovetailing" of the concepts to allow flexibility. There is no reason, for example, to exclude a child with AIDS and wasting syndrome from palliative care services because the child is receiving total parenteral nutrition even though the treatment might prolong the survival time of the child. Thoughtful considerations of this nature will serve to prevent the exclusion of many children from hospice services until the last minute when neither they nor their families can benefit from such services or they can no longer psychologically take advantage of palliative care. Although our referrals come mainly from acute care facilities, part of the process of determining suitability for admission is a careful assessment of the child's potential life expectancy. Because of our experiences with prolonged survival of children with certain supposedly "lethal" diagnoses, we have been personally assessing as many of these children as possible in their own facility prior to acceptance for admission.

One other important consideration involved in the determination of hospice needs of the child is the child's own preferences if known. This can be a difficult problem because it involves an assessment of the child's ability to understand the nature of death and dying, his or her religious beliefs and preferences, ability to deal with pain, and personal needs and relationships. Nevertheless in those situations where a child or young adolescent has sufficient awareness of their illness, I believe it is imperative to involve the child in the decision-making process with regard to such specifics as "Do Not Resuscitate" orders and treatment plans. Indeed, with regard to pain management, the child (who is experiencing the pain) should be the primary determinant of this process to the extent that they can be empowered to do so.

NEEDS THAT CANNOT BE ADDRESSED
IN HOME OR ACUTE CARE

Why then inpatient hospice? The answer is because there are considerations that cannot be addressed either in the acute care setting or in the home. The burden of nursing care can often be substantial to family members, and their ability to cope with the day-to-day physical and emotional burdens of such care can be overwhelming. Other factors include the presence of extensive pain requiring precarious dosages of pain-relieving medications, physical acuity beyond the resources of the home setting, and management of other symptoms (severe vomiting, dehydration, feeding problems, and technology dependence). Also, the type of inpatient setting must be appropriate to the physical and psychologic needs of the family and child. The availability of a variety of resources—home care, day care, long-term and acute inpatient treatment, and respite care—is an ideal to be reached in the management of children with terminal illness (Figure A.1). The Palliative Care Inpatient unit specifically addresses the needs of the more physically involved children who need a higher level of care than home or day care, but

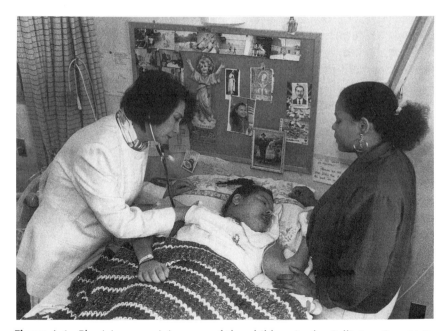

Figure A.1 Physician examining one of the children in the Palliative Care Unit, while the child's mother looks on. Saint Mary's Hospital for Children, with permission. (Courtesy of Carousel Studio, Bayside, NY)

who are not, by the terminal nature of their illness, appropriate for intensive care in an acute setting. To some extent, the decision concerning the appropriate setting for palliative care must depend on the coping mechanism of the family, as well as its ability to provide intensive nursing care in the home setting. The inpatient hospice program can address the psychologic and social needs of children and their families while providing the excellent nursing and medical care needed.

DECISION OPTIONS

The decision about where such services are provided is, of course, a decision that must be tailored to the individual and family needs. It will require a thorough understanding of the child's condition, both in terms of acuity of care and also prognosis, as well as an understanding of treatment options available. This type of decision making can at times bring out differences of opinion or emotion between families and caregivers and requires ongoing skillful reassessment of both fact and feeling. An example from our personal experience was an infant with a high thoracic meningomyelocele. After agonizing discussions with their neurosurgeon, the family elected to seek hospice care rather than elect surgery. The infant survived for several months, the meningocele healed spontaneously, and the child began to make developmental progress despite the presence of some degree of nonprogressive hydrocephalus. Some members of the treatment team were concerned that this infant was not truly a candidate for palliative care, but the family was convinced that their original decision was correct. The family was again referred to the neurosurgical team for reconsideration based on the changing status of the infant. Family members continued in their belief that they had made the correct decision and eventually the infant did indeed die of complications related to the underlying malformation. The care of this infant required careful, nonjudgmental assessment and reassessment, and a commitment on the part of the parents and the caretakers to the concept of palliative care. The family must be seen as an ongoing, active member of the treatment team whose participation and guidance in all treatment decisions is vital to the process.

DO NOT RESUSCITATE

Perhaps one of the most important decision options that many families face is the decision to request a Do Not Resuscitate (DNR) order. In our inpatient facility we have decided that a DNR order is a requirement at the time of admission. We have done this because we believe that the request of a DNR order gives us the reassurance that the family has come to an understanding of the terminal nature of the child's illness and is committed to allowing the child to die when the time comes. The DNR order, however, in no way precludes any other treatment options, even life-prolonging ones such as chemotherapy or total parenteral nutrition. New York State, along with others, has codified the circumstances under which an individual or family can request a DNR order. The circumstances defined in New York law are as follows:

1. The child has a terminal condition.
2. The child is permanently unconscious.
3. Resuscitation would be medically futile.
4. Resuscitation would impose an extraordinary burden on the patient in light of the patient's medical condition and the expected outcome of resuscitation for the patient.

Clearly these are broad definitions, which allow some degree of latitude in interpretation of the child's condition or status. The law further indicates the necessity of involving the child in the decision-making process, if the child is competent to make such a judgment. It does not specify an age at which such competence develops. The definition of competence then is left in the hands of a child psychologist, psychiatrist, or neurologist with expertise in this area. Nevertheless, it is important to explore with children to the extent that they are able the meaning of death, the concept of resuscitation, any religious or personal beliefs that might preclude such a request, as well as the child's feeling of individual autonomy. It helps where possible to involve the family in such discussions, as well as anyone else, for example, pastoral counselor, who might have a relationship with the child.

Since our inpatient facility is located in an independent skilled nursing facility for children, we are also often presented with the problem of transferring the patient to an acute care facility if necessary. Again, it must be emphasized that the DNR order does not preclude other treatment modalities that might be needed for palliative purposes, including under certain circumstances transfusions, intravenous antibiotics, chemotherapies, or other modalities that might require an acute care setting. When the child is transferred to an acute care setting, under the New York DNR law, the DNR order continues in effect for forty-eight hours after the transfer, unless discontinued (or renewed at the request of the family). This bridge is helpful for brief transfers, as the family does not have to be put through the rethinking process immediately during a potentially stressful period.

RESPITE

Although many families have requested inpatient services for their children during the terminal phase of their illness, others have opted for respite services for brief periods of time. These brief admissions are often requested at the time of a family emergency when resources need to be expended in dealing with that situation which may require travel or extended periods of time in a hospital. Sometimes requests are made for respite at the time of birth of a new baby in the family, and sometimes they are planned well in advance for a much-needed vacation. Because of the small size of our unit, it has been very difficult to provide respite care on an urgent basis but recent changes in regulations at the state level (New York) may allow us some flexibility by giving us the freedom to go over our bed allocation (provided space is available) to provide short-stay admissions for such emergencies. As mentioned earlier, our inpatient unit is part of a larger Palliative Care Program that involves both home care and day care services for terminally ill children. Careful integration with these programs assists us in the provision of planned inpatient respite admissions for those who can predict the need in advance. To effect this, representatives of the home care and day care programs are regular attendees at our admissions committee for the inpatient program, and are therefore continually updated on bed availability while the inpatient service is updated on the need for respite services in these programs.

PROCESS OF DEVELOPMENT

Before the development of our Palliative Care Program, a needs assessment was carried out. The study, which was done using data obtained from the New York City Health Department, indicated that there was a small but real need for pediatric hospice service in the New York area. The categories then defined were somewhat vague but subsequently we have been able to more precisely define the kinds of illnesses that could be cared for in a pediatric hospice program based on the kinds of referrals we have experienced. These included (1) Leukemia and Solid Tumors, Progressive Despite Conventional and/or Experimental Treatments; (2) Lethal Congenital Malformations (Brain, Cardiac, Renal, Pulmonary/Vascular, Hepatic); (3) Progressive Degenerative Neurological Disorders; (4) Progressive Neuromuscular Disorders; (5) Lethal Chromosomal Abnormalities; (6) Persistent Vegetative States; and recently (an unknown phenomenon at the time of the original feasibility study) (7) AIDS.

Although it was originally believed that the primary referrals would come from the category of incurable childhood malignancies, this has not turned out to be the case. The continuously improving outlook for childhood leukemia (the most common childhood malignancy) is one cause for this unexpected outcome. Also, the firmly established relationship between the treating oncologist and the families of children with malignancies often makes it difficult or impossible to make the referral to a palliative care facility in the terminal stage of such a prolonged illness. The most consistent referrals of malignant tumors is in the category of brain tumors (the second most common childhood malignancy), as the long-term outcome for many of these tumors is poor despite intensive research into modalities of treatment.

A repeated problem we have encountered is the issue of longevity within certain categories. For example, many of the so-called lethal congenital malformations and chromosomal disorders have allegedly brief life expectancies.[5-7] The obstetricians and pediatricians caring for these infants often dutifully inform the parents that their child has a life expectancy of days to weeks, and the families, based on this information, seek inpatient palliative services. Our experiences have often belied the "textbook" predictions of life expectancy; thus children with anencephaly, hydranencephaly, holoprosencephaly, and trisomy 13 have often lived for months or even years despite the uniformly poor outlook they allegedly have. Although no heroic measures are used to keep these children alive, it is our belief that good nursing care is the single strongest determinant in the real outlook for these children rather than the nature of the diagnosis per se. Even though this concept has never been explored on an experimental basis in pediatrics, at least two studies have demonstrated similar survival times in patients with Alzheimer's disease when provided with only good nursing care and no advanced technological support (including antibiotics and tube feedings), as opposed to those who were given such interventions.[8,9] We must, therefore, be quite circumspect when giving a prognosis of survival time based on the literature, since true survival may be as much a matter of the basic care provided as the nature of the illness or advanced technology.

DEFINING A SITE

The feasibility study mentioned above suggested several possible sites for a pediatric inpatient palliative care program including (1) the familiar inpatient acute care setting; (2) a separate facility within an acute care hospital where the needed caring and bereavement services could be provided; and (3) an existing skilled nursing facility with a dedicated unit where hospice services could be provided for children and their families. The acute care setting seemed to be more appropriate for a highly specialized unit that was dedicated to a specific disease type, such as a pediatric oncology program. However, because of the small numbers of children and the variety of categories of illness that might be cared for, it was recommended that our facility would best be served by a small (ten bed) expansion of our skilled nursing facility, and the development of a home care program of a somewhat larger size. The ten beds of the inpatient unit have been largely filled over the years, with 14 patients dying in the unit in 1991. Although the numbers of terminally ill children in the home care program varies considerably, the numbers have been increasing steadily, especially with the development of specific programs for children and families with AIDS. The number of children who died in the home care program in 1991 was 22. Since the original feasibility study estimated that there would be approximately 150 deaths per year of children who would be potentially hospice eligible in the Greater New York area, it appears that we are caring for approximately one-fifth of these children in our combined programs.

Considerations in the development of a pediatric palliative care program in a given community (other than the demographic considerations noted earlier) should take into account preexisting attitudes prevalent in the community, including those held by medical providers, and local political and social attitudes (such as the "not in my back yard" syndrome) that can plague unsuspecting agencies who might be caring for large numbers of AIDS victims, for example, as well as the problem of accessibility. The problem of accessibility has been particularly difficult for us at St. Mary's because, although we appear to be centrally located in the Greater New York area, the availability of conveniently located, safe, and affordable public transportation has been extremely limited for many families.

PHYSICAL CONSIDERATIONS AND DESIGN

We are very pleased with the design of our inpatient facility. Although it consists of one and two bedded rooms, the "treatment" area is much more like a large living room and there is plenty of space where the children, their families, and siblings as well as the staff and volunteers can congregate and interact. In essence, the homelike atmosphere of this facility is very different from the forbidding environment of most acute care facilities. The feeling engendered by the bright green colors and large airy skylights and windows overlooking Little Neck Bay causes most people who visit to feel very comfortable and invited, in contrast to the seemingly fear-engendering nature of the programs' purpose. The design seems to transport the individual from the hospital to the home giving an uplifting feel to the whole program. This feeling translates into better staff and patient acceptance of the facility and a great deal of family contact and interaction. Other suitable concepts could be developed, but the homelike nature of the structure should be emphasized and preserved.

REGULATORY INVOLVEMENT AND FUNDING

At a national level, pediatric palliative care programs remain an afterthought. The hospice regulations all relate to Medicare-eligible individuals, and none of our children are Medicare eligible. The focus on the geriatric population in this area is a manifestation of the effect of the huge difference in number of the elderly versus children faced with terminal illness. This fact has forced us to be creative in dealing with regulatory agencies, especially at the state and local levels. St. Mary's has been especially effective in working with the New York State Health Department to modify regulations that apply primarily to the geriatric population. We have worked very closely with the developers of the home care and skilled nursing facility regulators to make those programs available to the elderly apply and also fund programs for chronically and terminally ill children. In any locality, it will be imperative for the developers of children's hospice programs to become very knowledgeable about state and local regulations and funding sources for services to the geriatric population, especially those that govern Medicaid eligibility, and to work closely with the state regulating and funding agencies in order to secure appropriate modifications in regulations and funding sources, both public and private, to care for children. Since pediatric hospice programs require additional expenses (such as bereavement, education, and staff support programs) that are not usually reimbursed under skilled nursing or Medicaid sources, other funding from private philanthropic organizations and research grant programs must be vigorously pursued.

COMMUNITY AWARENESS AND INVOLVEMENT

Involvement of the community is essential to the success of any new program and getting the community interested involves a number of factors, not the least of which is recognition of the need for such a program. As previously mentioned, the general trend to deny the possibility of death in childhood given technical medical advances makes the job of getting support for such a program more difficult. Sometimes it takes a few courageous individuals who are personally aware of the need because of their own experience with the death of a child to challenge the complacency of the system. This has certainly been our experience, as such individuals have sought us out diligently from other parts of the country to assist them in the development of similar programs in other locales. But, individual experiences aside, the need to work with local community and consumer support groups is essential. The resources generated by these efforts include financial resources to provide "start-up" costs that are needed by any new program, but also a generally high profile in the community acts as a source of referral and reputation. Businesses and philanthropic organizations can also serve as sources of revenue for program development and building and renovating structures.

At times this issue of marketing and public relations can be difficult, especially in an area where privacy and confidentiality are so difficult to maintain, and where distortions can occur. An example of this pitfall came when, in the midst of a great deal of national publicity about our program, we realized that many people began to know St. Mary's only as a palliative care program; however, our mission was and is really much broader, and our palliative care program is only a small part of our total role. We were then in the position of having to redirect the orientation of the publicity to reflect our broader involvements and goals.

The issue of patient confidentiality is also of great importance. Although some families are very interested in assisting us in disseminating information about the program, others are rightfully concerned about the maintenance of their own privacy, and this must be honored completely if the institution hopes to remain respectable.

Other ways of developing community awareness include informational talks for professional organizations and hospital staffs. It is very important to get the medical community to understand the program in order to remind them that there are sources of help available during the trying times associated with the chronic and terminal illness of a child. The "Grand Rounds" presentation at the community hospital or teaching hospital can have a considerable effect on referral patterns and awareness of these services that may be needed only occasionally by individual practitioners.

Also other community resources should not be ignored. These include social and welfare agencies that often are aware of specific families and children in need, hospital discharge planners, as well as other community agencies such as home care programs, which may or may not provide either hospice services or services to children. These programs may not have the motivation to care for children or the expertise or resources to provide services to terminally ill children. Your program can then be a referral source for the adult program, or you can possibly work with them to develop the resources necessary to provide care for children as well.

STAFFING CONSIDERATIONS AND TRAINING OF CAREGIVERS

In many ways, the process of providing inpatient palliative treatment to children has been as much of a learning experience for us as a training experience. We knew we needed to recruit staff with a willingness to deal with the agonizing process of treating children with terminal illnesses and assisting their families through these difficult times, and yet there were few, if any, individuals experienced in this area. We needed to recruit a physician to direct the program, nursing personnel, child care technicians, social workers, and bereavement and pastoral counselors. These special people needed to understand the singular nature of the effect of a child's death on the family, the agonizing process of coming to grips with the terminal nature of the child's illness, the stages in this process for both the child and the family, and how to interact with the child and family in such a way as to provide support without becoming so involved as to need to seek support from the very families they were trying to assist. The amazing thing from my perspective is how willing most people are to learn under these circumstances as well as the very low turnover of personnel compared with other units within our institution.

Surely the physician primarily responsible for the care of these children must be sensitized to the special needs and problems faced by the many family members (parents, siblings, often grandparents, and others), as well as a sensitivity to the needs of the child. Consider the issue of pain management. Although there has been an explosion in research into pain evaluation and management in the past ten years, the problem of pain management in children remains a complex and confusing field.[10] The pediatrician who cares for these children must shed many of the traditional preconceptions of pain management in children (e.g., children don't experience pain as much as adults, or the child might become addicted to pain medication if it is given in adequate amounts). Although many younger pediatricians have been trained in this area, there is evidence that some continue to hold antiquated beliefs about pain management.[11]

Also, for the pediatrician, the problems of giving specific life expectancy predictions must be understood as previously mentioned. There are no training programs at present, to my knowledge, which provide both training and experience in this area and these programs must now be developed.

Similarly, special training for nursing personnel is also imperative. In any hospital setting, but especially in the palliative care setting, the nurse is the critical component in making the program work. The nurse is the frontline listener and observer of the child and family's needs. The nurse is there and must make complex decisions about care and management in critical moments. The nurse must provide simple nonjudgmental support and provide that support even when the family is in a confused or ambivalent state. The nurse must provide service coordination, and in many instances is called on to provide follow-up caring and support. Although much of the literature on pain evaluation is disseminated in pediatric nursing journals, hands-on experience in this difficult area is essential to the learning process.

Other nursing personnel, such as child care technicians and child care workers, also need special training and support in these areas. Some of the younger workers have difficulty dealing with larger issues, such as Do Not Resuscitate orders, confidentiality, and patient and family autonomy. Training programs for anyone involved in pediatric palliative care need to emphasize the importance of these concepts, as well as the basic methods of caring for chronically ill children.

The special needs of the families of these children also require special skills on the part of social workers and counselors involved in caring for these children and their families. The inclusion of social work students and pastoral care trainees has been one of the specially successful aspects of our inpatient program. Some students have shown a special interest in this field and have made significant contributions to our program while learning the specific skills needed for bereavement counseling and ongoing therapeutic intervention with the family of the dying child. Although long-term follow-up of the families of children who have died while in our care has been difficult (the old problem of funding again), we have nevertheless been able to provide a newsletter with contributions from many of the families over long periods of time, as well as a yearly memorial service and tree planting to which we invite the families of the children who have died while in our care. The large attendance at this program is a tribute to the long-term positive effects that the caring personnel have had on so many families.

SUPPORT OF CAREGIVERS

It is, of course, not sufficient to support only the families; we must provide ongoing training and support for the caregivers as well. The concept of a working team of caregivers is very useful in this context. The team can meet on patient-care issues, but it can also provide outlets for problems that arise on a continuous basis. The more experienced members of the team can provide insight into problems and those with special skills in counseling can help open up areas where fatigue and burnout may be entering the process. Difficult problems of identification, appropriate roles, and separation can be addressed. This process is very important because the nursing personnel and child care personnel play such an important frontline interface role with the children and their families. It is easy to underestimate the effects of continually dealing with families whose pre-existing psychologic and adjustment problems are compounded by the impending death of an infant or child. Here the resources of the psychiatrist, social worker, bereavement counselor, or pastoral counselor can often be quite helpful. The process requires continuing update and re-evaluation but it is well worth the investment in the ongoing effort to prevent the redevelopment of the barriers that I described earlier as the reason for my commitment to this program.

At this point I would like to mention the important role that volunteers have played in our program. We have noticed that the palliative care unit seems to attract many older, more mature volunteers . . . many who act as surrogate grandparents (Figure A.2). These individuals often have the ability to look beyond the prognosis and provide nurturing for the small children in an ongoing and deeply personal manner. They are often able to assist the children and families to accept the inevitable with simple warmth and kindness. They too, however, require continuing support and guid-

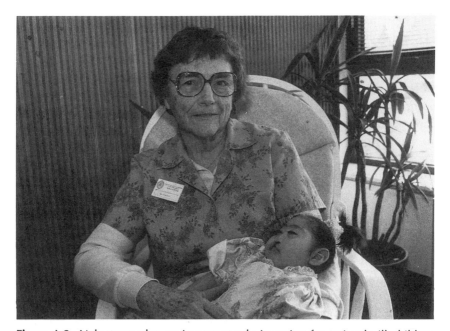

Figure A.2 Volunteers play an important role in caring for seriously ill children. Saint Mary's Hospital for Children, with permission. (Courtesy of Carousel Studio, Bayside, NY)

ance, especially in the areas of dealing with issues of closeness and separation.

BEREAVEMENT AND PASTORAL CARE

Bereavement services are an essential aspect of any palliative care program although the funding for such services is often not considered by regulatory bodies. Nevertheless it is important to provide a variety of services. Our program provides individual counseling, group counseling sessions, a newsletter, and memorial services, which are offered individually soon after the child's death and in the form of a larger service on a yearly basis. Small things, like a card at the time of the child's birthday, can also have a substantial impact. When possible, especially around the time of holidays, a phone call can also be greatly appreciated by the family. The yearly memorial service usually brings as many as 100 families even though we are only six years into the program.

Integral to the bereavement process is the acknowledgment of the individual family's religious faith and an understanding of the impact of beliefs about death and dying on the behavior and attitude of family members before and after the death of a child. Thus it is essential to have a well-integrated pastoral care program in place. At this time, the family members are often very aware of the feelings of fear, guilt, hostility, anger, and shame that they are experiencing. The pastoral counselor can help them acknowledge their feelings, affirm them, and then assist them in using their pre-existing religious beliefs to move on to more functional behaviors and social integration. For those with a strong belief system that includes a belief in the afterlife, the counselor can assist families in accepting that the pain they are experiencing is a phase and not a permanent state. For those families without a firm belief in the afterlife, the counselor can work with them in a more ethical mode of understanding that death will end the child's present pain and discomfort. When parents ask "How can God do this to my child?", the pastoral counselor can help put these questions into the context of the individual's belief system, thus preparing the groundwork for families to go beyond this situation and enter a more functional phase of life and behavior.

SUMMARY AND PERSPECTIVE

The inpatient component of the Palliative Care Program at St. Mary's Hospital for Children has now been in operation since 1985. Its development was an acknowledgment that there is a need for a place where children with terminal illnesses and their families can receive hospice services when they are unable to care for the child at home or the child's condition is no longer appropriate for an acute care setting. The experiences outlined here demonstrate that this setting can be effective for the compassionate treatment of dying children, providing them and their families with medical treatment, nursing care, pain management, respite when needed, emotional and psychological support, and bereavement and pastoral care services. The development, site selection process, physical environment, and interaction with regulatory agencies, funding sources, and community resources have been described. Training needs and staffing considerations and needs have been explored with the hope of indicating the need for more research and interest in these areas. Although this is a small program, it is a first in the field of palliative care in the United States. The inpatient unit is just one part of a larger effort including home care and day care programs designed specifically for a more rational approach to the care of the dying child than the nonapproach that existed when this pediatrician did his training. Our hope is to see the more general availability of such services in the future for those children and families in need.

Acknowledgments: The author acknowledges with gratitude, Burton Grebin, M.D.; Father Joel Harvey; Maud Reynolds, R.N.; Carmen Diaz-Sy, M.D.; Paul A. Klincewicz, M.S.W.; and Denise O'Connor.

NOTES

1. A comprehensive description of the initial development of this program has been previously presented by Dottie C. Wilson. Wilson, D.C. (1985). Developing a hospice program for children. In C.A. Corr and D.M. Corr (eds.), Hospice Approaches to Pediatric Care. New York: Springer, pp. 5–29.

2. Williams, W.C. (1984). The use of force. In R.C. Cole (ed.), The Doctor Stories. New York: New Directions, pp. 56–60.

3. Vianello, R., Lucamante, M. (1988). Children's understanding of death according to parents and pediatricians. J. Genet Psychol 149:305–316.

4. Emery, J.L. (1990). Attitudes of parents and paediatricians to a baby's death. J R Soc Med 83:423–24.

5. Baird, P.A., Sadovnick, A.D. (1984). Survival in infants with anencephaly. Clin Pediatr 23:268–71.

6. Pomerance, J.J., Morrison, A., Williams, R.L., Schifrin, B.S. (1985). Anencephalic infants: life expectancy and organ donation. J. Perinatol 9:33–37.

7. Pober, B.R., Greene, M.F., Holmes, L.B. (1986). Complexities of intraventricular abnormalities. J Pediatr 108:545–51.

8. Fabiszewski, K.J., Volicer, B., Volicer, L. (1990). Effect of antibiotic treatment on outcome of fevers in institutionalized Alzheimer patients. JAMA 263: 3168–72.

9. Riley, M.E., Crino, P. (1989). Eating difficulties in patients with probable dementia of the Alzheimer type. J Geriatr Psychiatry Neurol 2:188–95.

10. McGrath, P.A. (1989). Evaluating a child's pain. J Pain Symptom Manage 4:198–214.

11. Meehan, J. (1989). Pain control in the terminally ill child at home. Issues Compr Pediatr Nurs 12:187–97.

Children's Literature on Death

CHARLES A. CORR

There is now available a large and growing body of literature designed to be read by or with young readers concerning issues that are related to dying, death, and bereavement. Of course, the existing literature in this field is not completely exhaustive of every topic, point of view, reading level, or approach. That would be too much to expect when one takes into account the many ways in which humans encounter dying, death, and bereavement, and the numerous issues that arise from such contacts. But the existing literature for young readers in this subject area is already very rich and rewarding. A very diverse audience can profit from reading this literature including healthy children who are being introduced to issues of separation, loss, and sadness; children who are living with a chronic, life-threatening, or terminal illness; children who are grieving the loss of a significant person (e.g., grandparent, parent, sibling, or peer) or object (e.g., a pet) in their lives; and adults who wish to help such children.

The practical problem confronting an adult who wishes to draw on this body of literature is to select a few useful titles from a large variety of available resources. This section opens with guidelines as to how adults might use books of this sort with young readers. It then provides an annotated list in four age groupings, which describes 72 representative books for young readers and mentions 14 more. The final section identifies 7 books for adults, many of which contain suggestions as to how additional resources might be located.

SOME GUIDELINES FOR ADULTS

The following guidelines are suggested for adults in selecting and using books for or with young readers. These guidelines are meant to apply to any adult who seeks to use literature to help children in this subject area, whether that adult is a parent, teacher, counselor, or just an interested person.

1. *Evaluate the book yourself before attempting to use it with a child.* No book suits every reader or every purpose. Authors bring to their work their own points of view, choices about subject matter, and decisions about how to approach topics. Readers may or may not find that the work of a particular author is congenial to their perspectives or needs. It is not enough to find a book on loss or grief; one also wants to be comfortable with the information that it contains and the attitudes that it conveys. In most cases, it should only take a short time for an adult to determine whether a particular book is appropriate and satisfactory.

2. *Select titles, topics, and approaches that suit the needs of the individual young reader.* To be useful, any book must respond to the needs of a particular child. Ask what the child needs to gain from a book and then search for a title that serves those purposes.

3. *Be prepared to cope with limitations.* Each book has its own strengths and limitations. Almost always we must work with flawed materials. If so, we must be creative in adapting resources to purposes. For example, some books might describe a dead person as being "in heaven"; others might say that he or she is "a memory." Are either or both of these explanations acceptable? In *The Tenth Good Thing About Barney*, a pet cat who has died is said to be "in the ground and he's helping grow flowers" (Viorst, 1971; see below). Is that a good explanation? In *My Turtle Died Today* (Stull, 1964; see below), we are told that "you have to live a long time before you die." Is that true? Until the advent of the perfect book, we must be prepared to exploit the strengths of not-quite-prefect books and to cope with their concomitant limitations.

4. *Match materials to the capacities of the individual reader.* Often this requires little more than determining a child's reading or interest level. Sometimes a precocious child will require more advanced materials; in other instances, an older child may need to be directed to less challenging titles. Thus, the groupings that follow in this chapter should only be taken as preliminary clusters, not as fixed categories for all children in a particular age bracket. Reread guideline number 2. Children with special needs should be assessed with great care. For example, some older children whose reading abilities do not match their age might be invited to join a project in which they help an adult assess the suitability of simpler materials for younger readers.[1] In this way, they are designated as partners in a joint project with the adult and their own limited abilities are not directly challenged by materials that are too difficult for them.

5. *Read along with children.* Some books for very young readers may call for the assistance of an adult interpreter. Many books afford opportuni-

ties for rewarding interactions when they are shared by child and adult readers. Discussing a book together can create the "teachable moment" from which all can profit.[2] Children often appreciate the interest shown by an adult who takes time to share a good book with them. Adults, in turn, can learn more about a child's insights and concerns through the sharing process. Reading together a book about death and grief can sometimes make it possible for children and adults to support each other in coping with sadness.

PICTURE AND COLORING BOOKS FOR PRESCHOOLERS AND BEGINNING READERS

Bartoli, J. (1975). *Nonna*. New York: Harvey House. A boy and his younger sister have good memories of being with their grandmother on her swing and of her cookies. Wisely, they are permitted to participate in her funeral, the burial, and the division of her property among the members of her family so that each receives some memento of her life. A candid, attractive, and helpful story for young readers.

Boulden, J. (1989). *Saying Goodbye*. Santa Rosa, CA: Author. The story in this little book talks about death as a natural part of life, the feelings that are involved in saying goodbye, and the conviction that love is forever. The format is that of an activity book which allows the child-reader to draw pictures, color images, or insert thoughts on its pages. *Saying Goodbye* has won an award from the National Hospice Organization and is widely used in hospice and grief work with children. Available from the author at P.O. Box 9358, Santa Rose, CA 94505; tel. (707) 538-3797.

Brown, M. W. (1958). *The Dead Bird*. Reading, MA: Addison-Wesley. This early classic in the field offers an extremely simple, but attractive, text and pictures for very young readers. In a straightforward way, the story describes some children who find a wild bird that is dead in the woods. They touch the bird, bury it in a simple ceremony, and return to the site each day to mourn ("until they forgot"). Sadness need not last forever; life can go on again.

Buscaglia, L. (1982). *The Fall of Freddie the Leaf: A Story of Life for All Ages*. Thorofare, NJ: Slack. Photographs of leaves on a tree in the park are accompanied by a text in which one leaf (Freddie) asks another (Daniel) to explain their anticipated fall from the tree and the meaning of life. Fear of dying is compared to fear of the unknown and to natural changes in the seasons. Life itself is its own purpose and death is a kind of comfortable sleep. Adults will want to evaluate the messages in this book and confirm or correct what children might draw from them.

Clardy, A. F. (1984). *Dusty Was My Friend: Coming to Terms with Loss*. New York: Human Sciences. Benjamin (8) remembers his friend Dusty (10), who was killed in an automobile accident. Benjamin struggles to understand his feelings about losing a friend in this way. Benjamin's parents respond in helpful and informative ways. They give Benjamin permission to articulate his thoughts and feelings, to grieve for his loss, to remember the good times that he shared with Dusty, and to go on with his own life.

Cohn, J. (1987). *I Had a Friend Named Peter: Talking to Children About the Death of a Friend*. New York: Wm. Morrow. One section of this book is intended to prepare adults for the work of assisting children in coping with death. The children's section describes Beth's reactions when her friend, Peter, is killed by a car. Beth's parents and her teacher are portrayed as attentive and helpful in responding to Beth's needs, the needs of her classmates, and the needs of Peter's parents.

De Paola, T. (1973). *Nana Upstairs and Nana Downstairs*. New York: Putnam. Tommy likes to visit his grandmother and his great-grand-mother, the two nanas in the book's title. Tommy and his great-grandmother are especially close; they share candy, play with toys and imaginary beings, and both are restrained in their chairs in one picture. One morning, Tommy is told that Nana Upstairs is dead. He does not believe this until he sees her empty bed. A few nights later, Tommy sees a falling star and accepts his mother's explanation that it represents a kiss from the older Nana who is now "upstairs" in a new way. This interpretation has been criticized (Bernstein, 1983) as reinforcing undesirable childhood concepts of death, especially when an older Tommy repeats the experience and interpretation after the death of Nana Downstairs. A charming story about relationships, whose interpretations should be addressed with caution.

Dodge, N. C. (1984). *Thumpy's Story: A Story of Love and Grief Shared by Thumpy, the Bunny*. Springfield, IL: Prairie Lark Press (P.O. Box 699-B, 62705). Through text and pictures, Thumpy tells a story about the death of his sister, Bun, and its effect upon their family. Children relate easily to this simple story, which encourages them to share sadness and to go forward with living and loving. Also available in Spanish and as a coloring book. An accompanying workbook, *Sharing with Thumpy My Story of Love and Grief* (1985), allows children to draw and write about their own family and loss experiences.

Fassler, J. (1971). *My Grandpa Died Today*. New York: Human Sciences Press. David's grandfather tries to prepare the boy for his impending death. Among other things, he tells David that he does not fear death because he knows that David is not afraid to live. When he dies, David still needs to grieve. Nevertheless, David finds comfort in a legacy of many good memories from his relationship with his grandfather. And he is able to play again in just a little while because he knows that his grandfather would want him to do so. An example of how children often grieve in short spurts, perhaps as a defense against being overpowered by grief.

Harris, A. (1965). *Why Did He Die?* Minneapolis: Lerner. This book employs a question and answer format in which a mother explains death to her young son, Scott, as something that happens when someone's body, like an engine in a car, no longer works. The discussion is occasioned by the death of a friend's grandfather. Topics covered include aging, the life cycle, the fact that death in childhood is quite rare, memories, and quality of life.

Hazen, B. S. (1985). *Why Did Grandpa Die? A Book about Death.* New York: Golden Press. Young Molly and her grandfather have much in common. When Grandpa dies suddenly, Molly cannot accept that harsh fact. She feels awful and frightened, but she cannot cry. Molly's father reminds her that Grandpa was also his father and that he loved him very much, just as he knows that Molly did, too. As time passes, many things remind Molly of how much she misses Grandpa. After a long time Molly finally acknowledges that Grandpa will not come back and she cries over his death. But he still remains available to her through pictures, in her memories, and in stories shared with her family.

Heegaard, M. E. (1988). *When Someone Very Special Dies.* Minneapolis: Woodland Press (99 Woodland Circle, 55424; tel. (612) 926-2665). The storyline about loss and death in this little book provides inspiration and opportunity for children to illustrate and color. A useful vehicle for encouraging children to share thoughts and feelings. Two more recent (1991) publications of a similar sort by the same author are: *When Something Terrible Happens* and *When Someone Has a Very Serious Illness.*

Jordan, M. K. (1989). *Losing Uncle Tim.* Niles, IL: Albert Whitman & Co. This is an attractive and sensitive story about the friendship between a young boy and his Uncle Tim. Unfortunately, Uncle Tim becomes infected with the Human Immunodeficiency Virus (HIV), develops AIDS (Acquired Immunodeficiency Disease Syndrome), and dies. With the help of caring parents, the boy seeks solace through an idea that he had once discussed with his uncle: "Maybe Uncle Tim is like the sun, just shining somewhere else."

Kantrowitz, M. (1973). *When Violet Died*. New York: Parents' Magazine Press. After the death of Amy and Eva's pet bird, they have a funeral involving their young friends. The funeral includes poems, songs, punch, and even humor. The realization that nothing lasts forever makes everyone sad. But then Eva realizes that life can go on in another way through an ever-changing chain of life involving the family cat, Blanche, and its kittens.

Newman, K. S. (1988). *Hospice Coloring Book*. Orlando, FL: Hospice of Central Florida (2500 Maitland Center Parkway, Suite 300, 32751; tel. (407) 875-0028). Just what the title says it is.

Stickney, D. (1985). *Water Bugs and Dragonflies*. New York: Pilgrim Press. When a happy colony of water bugs notices that, every once in a while, one of their members seems to lose interest in their activities, climbs out of sight on the stem of a pond lily, and is seen no more, they begin to wonder what is happening. None of those who leave ever returns. So the members of the colony agree among themselves that the next to go will come back to explain where he or she had gone and why. The next climber broke through the surface of the water, fell onto a broad lily pad, and found himself transformed in the warmth of the sun into a dragonfly. One day the new dragonfly remembered his promise and tried to return, only to bounce off the surface of the water. He realizes that the members of the old colony might not recognize him in his new body, and he concludes that they will just have to wait for their own transformation in order to understand what happens. A booklet of faith in death as transformation.

Stull, E. G. (1964). *My Turtle Died Today*. New York: Holt, Rinehart & Winston. A boy seeks help for his sick turtle. His father suggests giving it some food, his teacher admits that she does not know what to do, and the pet shop owner says that the turtle will die. It does die and is buried. The boy and his friends discuss what all of this means and conclude that life can go on in another way through the newborn kittens of their cat, Patty. Much of this is sound, but the book also poses two questions that need to be addressed with care: Can you get a new pet in the way that one child has a new mother?; and Do you have to live—a long time—before you die?

Viorst, J. (1971). *The Tenth Good Thing About Barney*. New York: Atheneum. Barney, the boy's cat, dies, is buried, and is mourned. The boy's mother suggests that he might compose a list of ten good things about Barney to recite at the funeral. Among the items that the boy includes are these facts about Barney: he was brave and smart and funny and clean; he was cuddly and handsome and he only once ate a bird; it was sweet to hear him purr in my ear; and sometimes he slept on my belly and kept it warm. But that's only nine. Eventually, the tenth good thing is learned in the garden: "Barney is in the ground and he's helping grow flowers."

Warburg, S. S. (1969). *Growing Time*. Boston: Houghton Mifflin. When Jamie's aging Collie, King, dies, Jamie's father produces a new puppy. At first, Jamie is not ready for the new dog: premature replacement is a mistake. But after Jamie is allowed to express his grief, he finds it possible to accept the new relationship. Healthy grieving has its appropriate role in the lives of children and adults; it should not be suppressed.

Wilhelm, H. (1985). *I'll Always Love You*. New York: Crown. A boy and his dog, Elfie, grow up together. But Elfie grows old and dies while her master is still young. After her death, members of the family express regret that they did not tell her that they loved her. But the boy did so every night and realizes that his love for her will continue even after her death. He is not ready for a new puppy just now, even though he knows that Elfie will not come back and that there may come a time in the future when he will be ready for a new pet.

Zolotow, C. (1974). *My Grandson Lew*. New York: Harper. One night, 6-year-old Lewis wakes up and wonders why his grandfather has not visited lately. His mother says that Lewis had not been told that his grandfather had died four years ago because he had never asked. The boy says that he hadn't needed to ask; his grandfather just came. Son and mother share warm memories of someone they both miss: Lewis says, "he gave me eye hugs"; his mother says, "now we will remember him together and neither of us will be so lonely as we would be if we had to remember him alone."

STORYBOOKS AND OTHER TEXTS FOR PRIMARY SCHOOL READERS

Arnold, C. (1987). *What We Do When Someone Dies*. New York: Franklin Watts. This book combines a picture book format with informational content at about the level of primary school readers. Its scope covers feelings, concepts, and beliefs about death, but greatest attention is given to disposition of the body, funeral customs, and memorial practices.

Buck, P. S. (1948). *The Big Wave*. New York: Scholastic. Two Chinese boys are friends, Jiya the son of fishing people and Kino the offspring of poor farmers. After a tidal wave kills all the fishing people on the shore, Jiya mourns the loss of his family and chooses to live with Kino's warm and understanding family (vs. adoption by a rich man).

Years later, Jiya marries Kino's sister and chooses to move back to the seaside with his new bride. Loss is universal and inevitable, but life is stronger than death.

Bunting, E. (1982). *The Happy Funeral*. New York: Harper & Row. Can there be a "happy funeral"? Here, two young Chinese-American girls prepare for their grandfather's funeral. Food is provided for the journey to the other side, paper play money is burned, people cry and give speeches, a marching band plays, and a small candy is provided after the ceremony to sweeten the sorrow of the mourners. In the end, the children realize that, although they were not happy to have their grandfather die, his good life and everyone's fond memories of him did make for a happy funeral.

Carrick, C. (1976). *The Accident*. New York: Seabury. Christopher's dog, Bodger, is accidentally killed when he runs in front of a truck. Christopher goes over every detail of these events in an effort to overturn the loss. Christopher is angry at the driver, at his father for not getting mad at the driver, and at himself for not paying attention and allowing Bodger to wander to the other side of the road as they walked. Christopher's parents bury Bodger too quickly the next morning, before he can take part. But when he and his father are able to join together to erect a marker at Bodger's grave, anger dissolves into tears.

Coburn, J. B. (1964). *Annie and the Sand Dobbies: A Story About Death for Children and Their Parents*. New York: Seabury. Young Danny encounters death in two forms in this book: his toddler sister dies in her sleep of a respiratory infection and his dog runs away to be found frozen to death. A neighbor uses imaginary characters to suggest that the deceased are safe with God. A gentle, deeply spiritual book for primary school readers.

Coerr, E. (1977). *Sadako and the Thousand Paper Cranes*. New York: Putnam. This book is based on a true story about a Japanese girl who died of leukemia in 1955 as one of the long-term implications of the atomic bombing or Hiroshima (which occurred when Sadako was 2 years old). After her diagnosis, Sadako was in the hospital when a friend reminded her of the legend that the crane is supposed to live for a thousand years and that good health will be granted to a person who folds 1000 origami paper cranes. They began the task and Sadako's family members and friends helped. Sadako died before the project was finished, but her classmates completed the work and children all over Japan have since contributed money to erect a statue in her memory.

Corely, E. A. (1983). *Tell Me About Death, Tell Me About Funerals*. Santa Clara, CA: Grammatical Sciences. A funeral director describes a conversation between a young girl whose grandfather has recently died and her father. Topics include guilt, abandonment, and especially choices about funerals, burial, cemeteries, mausoleums, etc. Children are curious about such topics and will welcome this clear, noneuphemistic response. At one point, we are introduced to a child's delightful misunderstanding about the "polarbears" who carry the casket.

Donnelly, E. (1981). *So Long, Grandpa*. Trans. A. Bell. New York: Crown. Michael at 10 witnesses the deterioration and eventual death from cancer of his grandfather. The book portrays Michael's reactions and those of others. The way in which Michael's grandfather had helped to prepare the boy by taking him to an elderly friend's funeral is specially significant.

Goodman, M. B. (1990). *Vanishing Cookies: Doing OK When a Parent has Cancer*. Downsview, Ontario: The Benjamin Family Foundation (2401 Steeles Avenue West, Downsview, Canada M3J 2P1). Brightly colored illustrations alternate with text by a Canadian psychologist in this book for 7 to 12-year olds. The book is intended to bridge the gap between adults and children, and to help them share feelings in situations when an adult is coping with cancer. It encourages children to ask questions and provides information about cancer, treatments, coping with feelings, friends and school, and death. The title refers to the vanishing cookies that some children shared with their mother when they visited her in the hospital.

Greene, C. C. (1976). *Beat the Turtle Drum*. New York: Viking. Most of this book describes a loving, warm family which incudes 13-year-old Kate and 11-year-old Joss. When Joss is abruptly and unexpectedly killed in a fall from a tree, the family is flooded with grief. Conveying this sense of the many dimensions of bereavement is the book's strong point.

Johnson, J., & Johnson, M. (1978). *Tell Me, Papa: A Family Book for Children's Questions About Death and Funerals*. Omaha, NE: Centering Corp. Using the format of a discussion between children and a grandparent, this slim book provides an explanation of death, funerals, and saying good-bye. One of the many helpful resources available from the Centering Corporation (P.O. Box 3367, Omaha, NE 68103; tel. (402) 553-1200), who also publish *Hurting Yourself: For Teens Who Have Attempted Suicide* (1986).

Krementz, J. (1981). *How It Feels When a Parent Dies*. New York: Knopf. Short essays by 18 children and adolescents (7 to 16 years old) describe their individual reactions to the death of a parent. Each essay is accompanied by a photograph of its author. This book finds its strengths in its concrete realism and in the voices of its contributors.

Krementz, J. (1989). *How It Feels to Fight for Your Life.* Boston: Little, Brown; paperback edition by Simon & Schuster, 1991. Paralleling the previous entry, 14 youngsters (7 to 16 years old) describe their struggles with a wide variety of different life-threatening illnesses.

Lee, V. (1972). *The Magic Moth.* New York: Seabury. As a result of an incurable heart disease, 5-year-old Mark-O's 10-year-old sister, Maryanne, dies. Mark-O is helped to make sense of this experience by the metaphor of a moth which experiences a transition from one mode of life to another.

Miles, M. (1971). *Annie and the Old One.* Boston: Little, Brown. A 10-year-old Navajo girl is told that when her mother finishes weaving a rug it will be time for grandmother to return to Mother Earth. Annie tries to unravel the weaving in secret and to distract her mother from weaving, until the adults realize what is going on and her grandmother explains that we are all part of a natural cycle. When Annie realizes that she cannot hold back time, she is ready herself to learn to weave. The moral is that death is a natural part of life that need not be feared.

Peavy, L. (1981). *Allison's Grandfather.* New York: Chas. Scribners' Sons. Erica thinks about her friend Allison's grandfather (on his ranch) while he is dying. She asks the questions that we might all ask: Is he ready to die? Would she be told if her grandfather was dying? When Allison's grandfather does die, Erica's mother is there to hold his hand and to tell Erica about the experience.

Powell, E. S. (1990). *Geranium Morning.* Minneapolis: CarolRhoda Books. This is the story of two young children: Timothy, whose father died suddenly in an accident, and Frannie, whose mother is dying. The children struggle with strong feelings, memories, guilt ("if onlys"), and some unhelpful adult actions. But they also are helped by Frannie's father and by her mother before she dies. Above all, in sharing their losses, the two children help each other.

Simon, N. (1979). *We Remember Philip.* Chicago: Whitman. When the adult son of a male elementary school teacher dies in a mountain climbing accident, Sam and other members of his class can observe how Mr. Hall is affected by his grief. In time, Mr. Hall shares with the children a scrapbook and other memories of his son. Eventually, they plant a tree as a class memorial. An afterword addresses the fact that children often feel a sense of personal threat when death touches their lives or the lives of people close to them. They need opportunities to talk about their concerns, to share sadness, to gain reassurance, and to express compassion to those who care for them.

Smith, D. B. (1973). *A Taste of Blackberries.* New York: Scholastic. After the death of Jamie as a result of an allergic reaction to a bee sting, his best friend (the book's unnamed narrator) reflects on this unexpected event: Did it really happen or is it just another of Jamie's pranks? Could it have been prevented?; Is it disloyal to go on eating and living when Jamie is dead? The conclusions are that no one could have prevented this death, "some questions just don't have answers," and life can go on.

White, E. B. (1952). *Charlotte's Web*. New York: Harper. When this classic story was first published, the author was criticized for including death in a book for children. But he knew his audience better than his critics did. The story is mainly about friendship, on two levels: first, a young girl named Fern who lives on a farm saves Wilbur, the runt of the pig litter; later, Charlotte, the spider, spins fabulous webs which save an older and fatter Wilbur from the butcher's knife. In the end, Charlotte dies of natural causes, but her achievements and her offspring live on. Charlotte's death and threats to Wilbur's life do not traumatize young readers; instead, they are charmed and delighted.

Whitehead, R. (1971). *The Mother Tree*. New York: Seabury. Where do 11-year-old Tempe and her 4-year-old sister, Laura, turn for comfort in the early 1900s when their mother dies and Tempe is made to assume her duties? To a temporary spiritual refuge in the large, backyard tree of the book's title and eventually to good memories of their mother that endure within them.

LITERATURE FOR MIDDLE SCHOOL READERS

Arrick, F. (1980). *Tunnel Vision*. Scarsdale, NY: Bradbury. After Anthony Hamil hanged himself at 15, his family (Mom, Dad, Denise), friends (Carl, Ditto, and Jane), and teacher cope with feelings of bewilderment and guilt. There is no easy resolution for such feelings, but important questions are posed: What should be done in the face of serious problems?; Where should one turn for help?

Bernstein, J. E. (1977). *Loss: And How to Cope with It*. New York: Clarion. In a warm, knowledgeable, and helpful manner, this book advises young readers on how to cope with loss through death. Topics covered include: what happens when someone dies; children's concepts of death; feelings in bereavement; living with survivors; handling feelings; deaths of specific sorts of people (e.g., parents, grandparents, friends, pets); traumatic deaths (e.g., suicide or murder); and the legacy of survivors.

Blume, J. (1981). *Tiger Eyes*. Scarsdale, NY: Bradbury. When Davey's father is killed at the age of 34 during a holdup of his 7–11 store in

Atlantic City, the family must struggle with a difficult bereavement. Davey (15), her mother, and her younger brother all react differently and are unable to help each other. Seeking a change of scene, they travel to Los Alamos, the "bomb city," to visit Davey's aunt. They stay almost a year before finding better ways to mourn and decide to move back to New Jersey to pick up their lives once again. Important issues of safety and security, sharing with others, and being alone are explored in an insightful manner.

Cleaver, V., & Cleaver, B. (1970). *Grover*. Philadelphia: Lippincott. The facts are that when Grover was 11 his mother became terminally ill and then took her own life in order to spare herself and her family the ravages of her illness. From Grover's standpoint, the adults around him surround his mother's illness in mystery. After her death, his father cannot face the fact of her suicide or the depth of his grief. Instead, he tries to hold his feelings inside and to convince his son that the death was an accident. Thus, the issues posed by this fine story are: Whether or not one must endure life no matter what suffering it holds?; Is religion a comfort?; and How should one deal with grief?

Farley, C. (1975). *The Garden Is Doing Fine*. New York: Atheneum. Even while he is dying of cancer, Corrie's father inquires about his beloved garden. For her part, Corrie can neither tell him that the garden is dead nor can she lie. Instead, she searches for reasons that would explain why a good person like her father would die. She tries to bargain with herself and with God to preserve her father's life, until a wise neighbor helps her to see that, even though there may be no reasons, she and her brothers are her father's real garden. The seeds that he has planted in them will live on and she can let go without betraying him.

Grollman, S. (1988). *Shira: A Legacy of Courage*. New York: Doubleday. Shira Putter died at the age of nine in 1983 from a rare form of diabetes. Here the author tells Shira's story on the basis of her own writings and personal accounts from family members and friends. The effect is a celebration of life in which one finds hardship, courage, love, and hope.

Heegaard, M. E. (1990). *Coping with Death and Grief*. Minneapolis: Lerner Publications. Marge Heegaard experienced the death of her first husband when her children were 8, 10, and 12 years old. During the last 15 years she has worked as a grief and loss counselor with children and adults. This book describes change, loss, and death as natural parts of life, provides information and advice about coping with feelings, and suggests ways to help oneself and others who are grieving.

Jampolsky, G. G., & Taylor, P. (Ed.) (1978). *There Is a Rainbow Behind Every Dark Cloud*. Berkeley, CA: Celestial Arts. Eleven children, 8 to

19 years old, explain what it is like to have a life-threatening illness and the choices that youngsters have in helping themselves (e.g., when one is first told about one's illness, in going back to school, in coping with feelings, and in talking about death).

Jampolsky, G. G., & Murray, G. (Ed.) (1982). *Straight from the Siblings: Another Look at the Rainbow.* Berkeley, CA: Celestial Arts. Another book from the Center for Attitudinal Healing. Here the authors are brothers and sisters of children who have a life-threatening illness. Topics include the feelings of the siblings and ways to help all of the children who are involved in such difficult situations.

LeShan, E. (1976). *Learning to Say Good-By: When a Parent Dies.* New York: Macmillan. Numerous case histories are employed to describe experiences of grief following the death of a parent and ways in which adults often respond to children's mourning. Topics covered include overprotection, honesty and its importance, trust, sharing, funerals, fear of abandonment, anticipatory grief, and guilt, as well as recovering from grief, accepting the loss of the deceased, maintaining a capacity for love, and meeting future changes. A helpful book for children and adults.

Little, J. (1984). *Mama's Going to Buy You a Mockingbird.* New York: Viking Kestrel. Jeremy and his younger sister, Sarah, only learn that their father is dying from cancer by overhearing someone talking about it. Lack of information and limited contacts when he is in the hospital leave the children confused and angry. After the death, the children are permitted to attend the funeral, but it does not seem to have been a very helpful experience for them. Also, they must take on new responsibilities resulting from a relocation and their mother's return to school. All of this amply illustrates the many losses, large and small, that accompany dying and death. Another theme, the need for support from others, is evident in the relationships within the family and in Jeremy's new friendship with Tess, a girl who has been deserted by her mother and is treated like an outcast at school.

Mann, P. (1977). *There are Two Kinds of Terrible.* New York: Doubleday/Avon. Robbie breaks his arm, is hospitalized, and has an operation, but it ends. His mother develops cancer and dies, but the experience for Robbie and his "cold fish" father seems to have no conclusion. They are together, but each grieves alone until they begin to find ways to share their suffering and their memories. Good vignettes, e.g., a substitute teacher threatens to call Robbie's mother when he misbehaves.

Paterson, K. (1977). *Bridge to Terabithia.* New York: Crowell. 11-year-old Jess and Leslie have a special, secret meeting place in the woods, called

"Terabithia." But when Leslie is killed one day in an accidental fall on her way to visit Terabithia alone, the magic of their play and friendship is disrupted. Jess grieves the loss of this special relationship and is supported by his family. Eventually, he is able to initiate new relationships that will share friendship in a similar way with others.

Richter, E. (1986). *Losing Someone You Love: When a Brother or Sister Dies.* New York: G. P. Putnam's Sons. Fifteen adolescents describe in their own words how they are feeling in response to a wide variety of experiences of sibling death. Many young people will identify with what these teen contributors have to say and will find it important to know that they are not alone in their feelings of grief.

Rofes, E. E. (Ed.), and the Unit at Fayerweather Street School. (1985). *The Kids' Book about Death and Dying, by and for Kids.* Boston: Little, Brown. This book is the result of a class project involving a teacher and a group of 14 of his 11–14 year old students. It describes what these young authors have learned about a wide range of death-related topics: what is involved in a death; funeral customs; thoughts about the death of a pet, an older relative or parent, or a child; violent deaths; and whether there is life after death. The book makes clear what children want to know about these subjects and how they want adults to talk to them. The opening and closing chapters reflect on what is involved in learning to talk about death and on what has been learned in this project. One main lesson is that "a lot of the mystery and fear surrounding death has been brought about by ignorance and avoidance" (p. 111). Another lesson is expressed in the hope "that children can lead the way in dealing with death and dying with a healthier and happier approach" (p. 114).

Romond, J. L. (1989). *Children Facing Grief: Letters from Bereaved Brothers and Sisters.* St. Meinrad, IN: Abbey Press. After the death of Mark, her seven-year-old son, the author found herself obliged to help John, her three-and-a-half year old surviving son, cope with his brother's death. In listening to John's questions and comments, she began to record other observations of surviving siblings. In this slim book, the observations of 18 children (ages 6–15) are organized in the form of letters to a friend. Helpful comments from young people who have been there in grief.

Shura, M. F. (1988). *The Sunday Doll.* New York: Dodd, Mead. At the time of her thirteenth birthday, Emily is shut out by her parents from something terrible that is going on and that somehow involves her older sister Jayne (18). Emily is sent off to visit Aunt Harriet in Missouri, who had previously sent Emily an Amish doll without a face. Eventually, Emily learns that Jayne's boyfriend has been missing; later he is found to have taken his life. Meanwhile, Aunt Harriet suffers one of her "spells" (transient ischemia attacks) and comes close to death, but she also shows Emily her own strengths and that (like the Sunday doll) one can choose which face to present to the world. A richly textured story.

Sternberg, F., & Sternberg, B. (1980). *If I Die and When I Do: Exploring Death with Young People*. Englewood Cliffs, NJ: Prentice-Hall. This book is the product of a 9-week middle-school course on death and dying taught by the first author for three years in Colorado. The text mainly consists of drawings, poems, and statements by the students on various death-related topics, plus a closing chapter of twenty-five suggested activities.

LITERATURE FOR HIGH SCHOOL READERS

Agee, J. (1969). *A Death in the Family*. New York: Bantam. This novel won the Pulitzer Prize for, among other things, its unerring depiction of the point of view of two children in Knoxville, Tennessee, in 1915. When Rufus and his younger sister, Catherine, are told of the accidental death of their father, they struggle to understand what has happened and to grapple with its implications. Some questions are acceptable: Is death like waking up in heaven where the people on earth can no longer see you?; Do animals go to heaven, too? Other questions seem less appropriate to adults: What did it mean to say that God took their father to heaven because he had "an accident" ("not in his *pants*," Rufus wanted to tell Catherine)? And if their father was dead and they would never see him again, did that mean he would not be home for supper? When Rufus asks if they were "orphans," so that he could mention this one day in school to the other children, Catherine wonders what it is to be "a norphan." Adolescent and adult readers alike can learn much from Agee's portrait of the ways in which the children experience unusual events, sense strange tensions within the family, and strive to work out their implications.

Craven, M. (1973). *I Heard the Owl Call My Name*. New York: Dell. This novel describes a young Episcopal priest with a terminal illness who is sent by his bishop to live with Indians in British Columbia. The Indians recognize that death will come when the owl calls someone's name. From them, the bishop hopes that the young priest will learn to face his own forthcoming death.

Deaver, J. R. (1988). *Say Goodnight, Gracie*. New York: Harper & Row.

Jimmy and Morgan have been close friends since birth. When Jimmy is killed by a drunken driver in an automobile accident, Morgan is disoriented by the extent of her loss. She is unable to face her feelings, attend Jimmy's funeral, or speak to his parents. Understanding parents offer support and tolerate Morgan's withdrawal from the world. Eventually, a wise aunt (who is also a psychiatrist) helps Morgan confront her feelings in a way that leads her to more constructive coping and to decide to go on with living.

Greenberg, J. (1979). *A Season In-Between*. New York: Farrar. Carrie Signer, a seventh grader, copes with the diagnosis of her father's cancer in spring and his death that summer. Rabbinical moral: turn scratches on a jewel into a beautiful design.

Gunther, J. (1949). *Death Be Not Proud: A Memoir*. New York: Harper. One of the earliest books of its type, this is a moving account of a 15-month struggle with a brain tumor by the author's 15-year-old son.

Hughes, M. (1984). *Hunter in the Dark*. New York: Atheneum. Mike Rankin is going hunting in the Canadian woods for the first time. He has leukemia (and overprotective parents) and needs to face life and death on his own. In other words, this novel is about one adolescent's efforts to confront threats at different levels in his life.

Klagsbrun, F. (1976). *Too Young to Die: Youth and Suicide*. New York: Houghton Mifflin; paperback edition by Pocket Books, 1977. A simple, clear, informed, and readable introduction to the myths and realities surrounding youth suicide, with useful advice for helpers. There are many other books for young readers in this subject area, such as: W. Colman, *Understanding and Preventing Teen Suicide* (Chicago, Children's Press, 1990); D. B. Francis, *Suicide: A Preventable Tragedy* (New York: E. P. Dutton, 1989); S. Gardner & G. Rosenberg, *Teenage Suicide* (New York: Messner, 1985); M. O. Hyde & E. H. Forsyth, *Suicide: The Hidden Epidemic* (New York: Franklin Watts, 1986); M. & J. Johnson (see entry above); J. Kolehmainen & S. Handwerk, *Teen Suicide: A Book for Friends, Family, and Classmates* (Minneapolis: Lerner, 1986); J. Langone (see next entry); J. M. Leder, *Dead Serious: A Book for Teenagers about Teenage Suicide* (New York: Atheneum, 1987); and J. Schleifer, *Everything You Need to Know About Teen Suicide* (rev. ed.; New York: The Rosen Publishing Group, 1991).

Langone, J. (1986). *Dead End: A Book about Suicide*. Boston: Little, Brown. John Langone is a medical reporter who has published other books (*Death is a Noun: A View of the End of Life*, 1972; *Vital Signs: The Way We Die in America*, 1974) for mature young readers about death in our society. Langone's work on suicide is current, thoughtful, detailed, and particularly well-suited for the education of teenage readers.

Lewis, C. S. (1976). *A Grief Observed*. New York: Bantam. This British author is well known for the *Screwtape Letters, Tales of Narnia*, and learned treatises in Christian theology. Lewis married rather late in life an American woman who soon developed cancer and died. This book reflects the author's efforts to record his own experiences of grief on notebooks that were lying around the house. The result is an unusual and extraordinary document, a direct and honest expression of one individual's grief which has helped innumerable readers by normalizing their own experiences in bereavement. A brief introduction establishes the context.

Martin, A. M. (1986). *With You and Without You*. New York: Holiday House; paperback by Scholastic. This book is about the reactions of parents and four children in a family when the father is told that he will die in the next 6 to 12 months as a result of an inoperable heart condition. Each member of the family tries to make the father's remaining time as good as possible. After his death, they struggle to cope with their losses. One important lesson is that no one is ever completely prepared for a death; another is that each individual must cope in his or her own way.

Pendleton, E. (Comp.) (1980). *Too Old to Cry, Too Young to Die*. Nashville: Thomas Nelson. Pendleton is described as the compiler of this book, in which 35 teenagers describe their experiences in living with cancer. The voices of these adolescent authors ring with truth about such topics as treatments, side effects, hospitals, parents, siblings, friends, etc.

Tolstoy, L. (1960). *The Death of Ivan Ilych and Other Stories*. New York: New American Library. The title story of this collection is an exceptional piece of world literature, first published in 1886. Ivan Ilych is a Russian magistrate who drifts into marriage (mainly for social reasons), enjoys playing cards with his friends, and in all else prefers to confine himself to what might be written down on letterhead stationery. In the prime of life, Ivan is afflicted with a grave illness which becomes steadily more serious. As his health deteriorates, Ivan suddenly realizes that glib talk in college about mortality does not just apply to other people or to humanity in general. Those around Ivan gradually withdraw and become more guarded in what they say to him, except for one servant and his young son. A masterful portrait of the experience of dying.

FOR ADULTS: FURTHER GUIDELINES AND RESOURCES

Old books go out of print, even as new books come into print. A good book for children that is currently out of print is still likely to be available in public libraries or in learning resource centers in the schools. Other titles can be identified through ongoing bibliographical guides, as well as through the following resource volumes.

Bernstein, J. E., & Rudman, M. K. (1989). *Books to Help Children Cope with Separation and Loss*, Vol. 3. New York: R. R. Bowker. Vols. 1 & 2 were authored by Bernstein alone and published, respectively, in 1977 & 1983. These three volumes contain informed and sensitive descriptions of a very large number of books for children. They are characterized by broad topical range and keen evaluations. The author(s) advocates and explains at length the concept of bibliotherapy, the use of books to help children cope with loss and grief. Indispensable guides and reference tools.

Corr, C. A., & McNeil, J. N. (Eds.) (1986). *Adolescence and Death*. New York: Springer Publishing Co. Addresses death, dying, bereavement, and suicide in the world of adolescents, together with constructive suggestions for parents, counselors, and educators. Also contains annotated guides to literature for young people and for adults.

Grollman, E. A. (1990). *Talking About Death: A Dialogue Between Parent and Child* (3rd ed.). Boston: Beacon Press. There are four major sections in this book: a set of principles for helping children to cope with death; a passage which an adult should read along with a child; a lengthy guide to responding to questions that may naturally arise in the read-along section; and a guide to helpful resources. A classic in this field.

Wass, H., & Corr, C. A. (Eds.) (1984). *Childhood and Death*. Washington, DC: Hemisphere. A major resource in its field, with chapters on helping children at home, in the schools (both at the primary and secondary levels), while they are dying, or when they are bereaved, plus lists of selected, annotated resources (books for adults, books for children, organizations, and audiovisuals).

Wass, H., & Corr, C. A. (Eds.) (1984). *Helping Children Cope with Death: Guidelines and Resources* (2nd ed.). Washington, DC: Hemisphere. Four chapters offer guidelines for parents and others who seek to enter the world of a child who is coping with death, plus three chapters of annotated resources (printed materials, audiovisuals, and organizations).

Wass, H., et al. (1980 & 1985). *Death Education: An Annotated Resource Guide*, Vols. I & II. Washington, DC: Hemisphere. Annotated bibliographies of various sorts of resources, including children's literature in Vol. II.

Wolfelt, A. (1983). *Helping Children Cope with Grief*. Muncie, IN: Accelerated Development. Advice, suggested activities, and resources for helping grieving children.

NOTES

1. Lamers, E.P. (1986). Books for adolescents. In C.A. Corr and J.N. McNeil (Eds.), Adolescence and Death. New York: Springer, pp. 233–242.

2. Carson, U. (1984). Teachable moments occasioned by "small deaths." In H. Wass and C.A. Corr (Eds.), Childhood and Death. Washington, DC: Hemisphere, pp. 315–343.

ADDITIONAL RESOURCES

Activity Books for Children

Bignano, Judith. *Living with Death: Journal Activities for Personal Growth, Gr 5–9*, Carthage, IL: Good Apple, Inc., 1991. $6.95.

Cora, Mary Jane. *Living with Death: Activities to Help Children Cope with Difficult Situations, GR 1–4*, Carthage, IL: Good Apple, Inc., 1991. $6.95.

Heegard, Marge. *When Someone Has a Very Serious Illness*, Minneapolis: Woodland Press, 1991. Distributed by The Rainbow Connection, Burnsville, NC. $5.95.

Heegard, Marge. *When Someone Very Special Dies*, Minneapolis: Woodland Press, 1988. Distributed by The Rainbow Connection, Burnsville, NC. $5.95.

Loma Linda Hospice. *Someone Special Died: An Activity Book for Children Experiencing the Loss of a Loved One*, Loma Linda, CA: Loma Linda Hospice, 1990. $5.

Resources for Educators

American Federation of Teachers. *The Medically Fragile Child in the School Setting*, Washington, DC: American Federation of Teachers, AFL-CIO, 1992. Item #451, $5.

Berry, Joy. *About Traumatic Experiences*, Chicago: Children's Press, 1990. Distributed by the Rainbow Connection, Burnsville, NC. $4.95.

Blackburn, Lynn. *The Class in Room 44*, Omaha: Centering Corporation, 1991. $3.50.

Braden, Majel. *Grief Comes to Class*, Omaha: Centering Corporation, 1992. $4.25.

Corr, C. A. and J. N. McNeil. *Adolescence and Death*, New York: Springer, 1986.

Fox Valley Hospice. *Child Grief: A Teacher Handbook*, Batavia, IL: Fox Valley Hospice, 1987.

Gordon, A. K. and D. Klass. *They Need to Know: How to Teach Children About Death*, Englewood Cliffs, NJ: Prentice-Hall, 1979.

Huntley, Theresa. *Helping Children Grieve*, Minneapolis: Augsburg Fortress, 1991. Distributed by The Rainbow Connection, Burnsville, NC. $6.95.

Jewette, Claudia. *Helping Children Cope with Separation and Loss*, Harvard, MA: The Harvard Common Press, 1982.

LeGrand, L. E. *Coping with Separation and Loss As a Young Adult*, Springfield, IL: Charles C. Thomas, 1986.

Lonetto, Richard. *Children's Conceptions of Death*, New York: Springer, 1980.

Mellonie, Bryan and Robert Ingpen. *Lifetimes: The Beautiful Way to Explain Death to Children, PreK–Gr 4*, New York: Bantam, 1983. Distributed by Centering Corporation, Omaha, NE. $8.95.

Murphy, Eva, (ed). *Books and Films on Death and Dying for Children and Adolescents: An Annotated Bibliography*, Boston: The Good Grief Program, 1988. $10. Updated supplement also available.

National Cancer Institute. *Students with Cancer: a Resource for the Educator*, Bethesda, MD: National Cancer Institute, 1984.

Ragouzeos, Bobbe. *The Grieving Student in the Classroom: Guidelines and Suggestions for Classroom Teachers and School Personnel of Grades K–12*, Lancaster, PA: Hospice of Lancaster County, 1988. $2.75.

Russell, Kate. *Guiding Children Through Grief*, Omaha: Centering Corporation, 1989. $5.25.

Seibert, Dinah; Drolet, Judy; and Joyce Fetro. *Are You Sad Too? Helping Children Deal with Loss and Death*. Santa Cruz: E. T. R. Associates, 1993.

Wass, Hannelore and Charles Corr, (eds.). *Helping Children Cope with Death: Guidelines and Resources*, 2nd. ed. New York: Hemisphere Publishing Corporation, 1984.

Wolfelt, Alan. *Helping Children Cope with Grief*, Muncie, IN: Accelerated Development, Inc., 1983. Distributed by The Rainbow Connection, Burnsville, NC. $15.95.

Professional Journals

Death Studies
Hannelore Wass, ed.
Hemisphere Publishing Corporation
1010 Vermont Ave.
Washington, DC 20005

Loss, Grief, and Care: A Journal of Professional Practice
Haworth Press
28 W 22 St.
New York, NY 10010-6194

Omega
Robert Kastenbaum, ed.
Baywood Publishing Co.
Farmingdale, NY 17735

Suicide and Life-Threatening Behavior
American Association of Suicidology
Human Sciences Press
72 Fifth Ave.
New York, NY 10011

Thanatos
Florida Funeral Directors Services
502 E Jefferson St.
Tallahassee, FL 32314

Grief Periodicals for Adults and Children

Bereavement: A Magazine of Hope and Healing
Andrea Gambell, editor
350 Gradle Dr.
Carmel, IN 46032

Fernside Inside
Newsletter of the Fernside Center for
    Grieving Children
P.O. Box 8944
Cincinnati, OH 45208
(513) 321-0282

The Forum Newsletter
Albert Lee Strickland, editor
Association for Death Education and Counseling
533 Stagg Lane
Santa Cruz, CA 95062
(408) 475-6527

Just for Us: A Bereavement Newsletter
    for Children and Teens
St. Mary's Hospital for Children
29-01 216th St.
Bayside, NY 11360
(718) 281-8000

Resource Distributors

Centering Corporation
1531 N Saddle Creed Rd.
Omaha, NE 68104-5064
(402) 553-1200

Compassion Book Service
479 Hannah Branch Rd.
Burnsville, NC 28714
(704) 675-9670

The Good Grief Program
Judge Baker Children's Center
295 Longwood Ave.
Boston, MA 02115
(617) 232-8390

Medic Publishing Company
P.O. Box 89
Redmond, WA 98073
(206) 881-2883

Mount Ida College
National Center for Death Education
777 Dedham St.
Newton Centre, MA 02159
(617) 969-7000, x 249

The Rainbow Connection
477 Hannah Branch Rd.
Burnsville, NC 28714
(704) 675-5909

Professional Associations

Association for Death Education and Counseling
Association Resources
638 Prospect Ave.
Hartford, CT 06105

The Center for Death Education and Research
1167 Social Science Bldg.
University of Minnesota
Minneapolis, MN 55455

The Foundation of Thanatology
630 W 168th St.
New York, NY 10032

American Associaton of Suicidology
2459 S Ash St.
Denver, CO 80222

INDEX

Acquired immunodeficiency syndrome
(AIDS). *See* HIV infection and
AIDS
Admission criteria
Edmarc Hospice for Children, 220–22
evaluation for hospital program,
250–51
Home Care for Children with Cancer
Project, 233, 234–36
Adolescent
developmental tasks of, 65–68
HIV infection and AIDS, 90–91
response to dying, 71–73, 97
AIDS. *See* HIV infection and AIDS
Analgesic interventions, 45–54. *See also*
Pain control
adjuvant therapy, 53–54
ladder for management, 46 (table)
Anxiety, 31

Baby Doe Regulations, 77–79
Bereaved parents. *See* Parents, bereaved
Bereavement. *See also* Grief
divorce and, 165–66
hospital program, 263
intervention goals, 129–33
after death, 131–33
before death, 129–30
intervention models and strategies,
133–38
grief counseling, 135–36
grief counseling, couples, 134–35
grief counseling, individual, 134
sibling, 140–53
support groups, 136–38, 161–62
Burnout, avoidance strategies for staff,
195–96

Camp Nabe, 162
Cardiorespiratory distress, 31–32. *See
also* Symptom control
Children and Grief: Living with Loss,
162–63

Clinical management issues
child's understanding of death, 9–21
HIV infection and AIDS, 85–104
neonatal death, 75–84
pain and symptom control, 22–59
psychosocial aspects, 60–74
Codeine, 49. *See also* Pain control
Communication, with dying child, 18–20
guidelines for, 19–20
techniques
nonverbal, 19
verbal, 68–69
Constipation, 32
Contractures, 35–36

Death
activities after, 118–19
child's understanding of
cognitive, 9–10, 15, 69
concepts of, 10–14
contributing factors, 14–17
developmental tasks, 60–68
phases of, 12–14
dignity and, 25
education, 154–57, 266–84
HIV infection/AIDS and, 100
literature on. *See* Literature on death
neonatal. *See* Neonatal death
preparation for, 69–71, 116–17
prior experience with, 15–16
process of, 54–55
social context of, 17–18
family culture, 18
global culture, 17
Decision making
DNR order, 253–55
hospital program and, 252–53
neonatal death and, 77–80, 108
Baby Doe Regulations, 77–79
family concerns, 79–80
financial concerns, 80
medical considerations, 77
selection and hospice, 110–11